SIMPLY ARMENIAN

Naturally Healthy Ethnic Cooking Made Easy

Also by **Barbara Ghazarian**

Descendants of Noah: Stories of Armenian Apostolic
Faith and Heritage

Also by **Mayreni Publishing**

My Patriarchal Memoirs
Armenians in the Ottoman Empire: An Anthology of Transformation–
13th-19th Centuries
A Village Remembered: The Armenians of Habousi
Boghos Nubar's Papers and the Armenian Question: 1915-1918

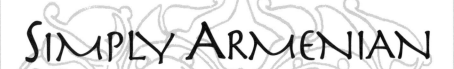

SIMPLY ARMENIAN

Naturally Healthy
Ethnic Cooking Made Easy

BARBARA GHAZARIAN

Mayreni Publishing • Monterey, California • 2004

Mayreni Publishing, Inc.
P.O. Box 5881
Monterey, California 93944

Simply Armenian: Naturally Healthy Ethnic Cooking Made Easy.
Copyright @ 2004 by Barbara Ghazarian

Printed in the United States of America

Library of Congress Control Number: 2003112820
Ghazarian, Barbara
Simply Armenian: Naturally Healthy Ethnic Cooking Made Easy
Includes index.

ISBN 1-931834-06-7

1. Cookery, Armenian. 2. Cookery, Middle East.

Special bulk-order discounts are available on this and other Mayreni Publishing books. Companies and organizations may purchase books for premiums or resale by contacting the Marketing Director at the address above.

Cover: Fresh quinces and Quince Preserves (page 266)
Bulgur Pilaf (page 59)
Shish Kebab (page 143)
Oldways' Mediterranean Diet Pyramid courtesy of
Oldways Preservation & Exchange Trust (http://oldwayspt.org)
All other illustrations are extracts from Armenian manuscripts reproduced from
the book, *Armenian Decorative Art* (Yerevan, 1955).

For Vatche and Talin

CONTENTS

SWEETS   233

GLOSSARY & INDEX   279

ACKNOWLEDGMENTS

Preparing this recipe collection for publication required years of sustained passion and persistence, and not just my own.

My deepest gratitude to—

Carolyn North Haley, my friend and writing companion, for her skillful and relentless editing of draft after draft of this manuscript. Carolyn, I could not have accomplished this book without your expertise.

My mother-in-law, Ashkhen Ghazarian, who journeyed to the United States to help me as a new bride and mother and who, despite the barrier of language, shared her legendary kitchen wisdom and recipes with me. *Tserkt talar, Medz Mama.*

The memory of my dear grandmother, Irene (Malkasian) Mooradian, whose gardening, cooking, canning, pickling, and strong ties to the age-old culinary traditions of Turkish Armenia provided the foundation and inspiration for this collection.

My cousin, Craig Wallen, whose love and knowledge of the food of our shared ancestry equals my own, and whose suggestions were invaluable to the successful adaptation of so many of these recipes to the contemporary kitchen while preserving the tastes, textures, and smells of our grandmother's table. Thank you, Craig.

My family of friends, especially Rhonda Redden, Debbie Weiner-Soule, Lisa Fucile, and Diane Kelly for listening to me, for brainstorming with me, and for supporting and encouraging me even when I went my own way.

Betsy Gould for paying attention to the final details.

My mother, Mary (Unsworth) Mooradian, whose adventurous spirit in the kitchen during her active life inspired me to explore this culinary path and whose generous legacy afforded me the opportunity to bring this book to fruition.

Lastly, I offer special gratitude to my husband and my daughter. You are my cheering section, and I am humbled by your love.

ARMENIAN COOKING MADE EASY

One of the greatest gifts Armenians have given the world is their cuisine. The Armenian table is magic, the cook a magician. The food is simple and easy to prepare, naturally healthy, and abundant.

The journey into a foreign cuisine is not necessarily an easy one. Armenian cooking can be intimidating for the novice, especially the non-Armenian spouse or the average American with an interest. I know—I'm one of you.

By descent, I am half Armenian on my father's side and a quarter Irish–quarter English on my mother's side. Except for every-other-weekend visits to my paternal grandparents and cousins who lived in the tight-knit Armenian immigrant community of Whitinsville, Massachusetts, I grew up a product of the public schools in a well-to-do insurance suburb of Hartford, Connecticut.

Then I fell in love with and married a very special Armenian man born in Aleppo, Syria.

Very quickly I realized that my husband, like most husbands no matter what their nationality, preferred the tastes and combination of foods traditional to his mother's kitchen. Motivated by a hope of pleasing the man I love and my new family of relatives, I began to explore the cuisine of our shared ancestry.

I soon discovered that some of the ingredients (bulgur and lentils), food combinations (stuffing vegetables with rice), and common practices (like drenching oven-hot baked pastry with cool, slightly flavored thick sugar syrup) upset my "red, white, and blue" sensibilities. I found recipe instructions often skimpy, and the use of untranslated foreign words rather than their English equivalents confusing. Also daunting was the intensive labor and time needed to prepare many of the traditional dishes.

In spite of these hurdles, or maybe because of them, I learned, and I wrote this book so that your exploration of this fabulous cuisine will be easier than mine, and your results more assured.

I have taken the intimidation factor out of Armenian fare, but not the taste, smells, and exotic look of the food. Nor have I made it fancy. For centuries, Armenians have been eating like sultans on what others considered scraps and pantry basics. Now you can, too.

While the culinary activities of the past are of great value and keep us in harmony with the earth, the seasons, and our humanity, for most of us foraging for wild grape leaves may be impractical in the 24/7 plugged-in workaday world we live in today. So, while the majority of the recipes included in this collection are authentic, all have been chosen and retooled to be simple, fast, and easy—even for an inexperienced cook. They have been tested and retested to ensure success, and if the flavors and textures of a dish can be reproduced using prepared foods or new technologies, I use them.

Most of the ingredients are readily available, and when they're not, I usually suggest a substitution. Uncommon ingredients are defined in the Glossary and can be purchased from the mail-order sources listed in the back of the book—no matter where you live in the United States.

Along my journey of discovery into the sensuous kitchen of my Armenian ancestry, many cooks shared their wisdom with me, and I have taken care to credit the originator of a particular recipe when appropriate. The handful of recipes that are my own improvisations, like my Chocolate Chip Choreg (page 212), are identified as well.

Whether you are a seasoned chef with many Middle Eastern cookbooks on your shelf, or you are new to the cuisine, this book is for you. My easy-to-follow instructions and delicious, fail-proof dishes will wow your family and friends, without your having to labor for days or spend a fortune to accomplish the task.

ABOUT THE FOOD

Rather than rely on condiments, sauces, or lots of seasonings, Armenian dishes depend upon the food itself, or the combination of foods, to give fine flavor. The cuisine relies heavily on bulgur (cracked wheat) and lentils for bulk and substance. Lots of vegetables extend the dishes, which are eaten with large quantities of bread, especially flatbread. Other than salt and black pepper, cayenne (hot red pepper) and cumin are the spices most often used.

Although *Simply Armenian* is not a vegetarian cookbook, many of the recipes are meat-free. This bias is due to historical influences. First, traditionally, Armenians farmed the soil or tended orchards. Second, for nearly two millennia Armenians have been Christians, and the Armenian Orthodox calendar has more than 180 fasting days a year! On those days, the faithful are asked to abstain from eating dishes containing animal products, including dairy. While few people follow the church calendar today, many do observe the dietary restrictions during Lent. For that reason, the Lenten dishes are marked (✍) for easy identification, and substitutions (no animal products) are noted when necessary.

Traditionally, lamb is the preferred meat. Beef can be substituted throughout the book, and beef is the meat of preference for most Armenians born in the Middle East because they say the lamb available there "smelled" odd. Chicken is a staple. Fish is infrequent; Armenians have historically been a landlocked people. Eggplant is a favorite. Nuts and fruits are used in everything.

Fresh fruit and cheese are usually the first dessert and are often offered as an appetizer, too. Meals end with strong coffee that packs a higher-octane punch than Italian espresso, and perhaps a world-class Armenian brandy or cognac. Sweets are traditionally served to guests at teatime and on holidays.

The ingredient most unique to this collection may be quince. Quince is a fruit related to apples and pears. It is native to the Caucasus and northern Persia (now Iran) and has been cultivated throughout the Mediterranean basin for centuries, but because it is rarely eaten raw, it has not been commonly used in the United States. But Armenians are a resourceful people known for their thrift and ingenuity, and my aunt had three quince trees growing in her yard. So, true to my grandmother's nature, she harvested those quinces every year and added quince dishes to our family's table.

My grandmother used to say, "Feed the body, so the soul can sing." Like thousands of Armenian cooks before her, and those of us who are following in her footsteps, it's time to learn the magic of creating a feast out of a basket of fresh vegetables and a handful of bulgur.

Armenian cuisine is a celebration of abundance, even in times or places of misfortune. It's time. Let's celebrate!

OVER A CENTURY IN AMERICA—
A CULINARY MEMOIR

More than anything, *Simply Armenian* is a collection of recipes that honors a kitchen and a cuisine based on relationships. Whether by birth or through marriage or by likenesses and similarities acquired by living next door to Turks, Persians, Syrians, Lebanese, Egyptians, Greeks, French, Russians, Georgians, Jews, or Americans for generations, the Armenian kitchen is a kindred kitchen.

Since ancient times, Armenians have lived on the land that today is eastern Turkey, northwestern Iran, and the southern Caucasus. According to legend and scripture, Noah's Ark came to rest atop Mount Ararat, the highest point in historic Armenia. By the late 19th century, when this memoir begins, my ancestors—like many Armenian ancestors—farmed historic Armenian soil in Armenian-populated towns and villages as Christian minority subjects of the Ottoman Empire.

My family is from the village of Pazmashen (Buzmashen in Turkish). In 1896, the Ottoman Turks, who had ruled the Armenians for six centuries, attacked the village. That killing spree, one of the worst of many massacres over generations, orphaned my grandfather, Eli (Yeghia) Mooradian, as a young child. It also catalyzed the elders of the village into action. My maternal great-grandfather, Sarkis Malkasian, was one of three young men selected by the village elders to travel to America to explore opportunities.

After landing in New York, my great-grandfather Sarkis made his way to the New England mill town of Whitinsville, Massachusetts. Whitinsville was already home to a small but growing number of Armenians (many from Pazmashen) who had found jobs in the huge, prosperous Whitin Machine Works foundry. My great-grandfather, too, went to work in the foundry.

By 1907, he had saved enough money to send for his wife, Behar (Sahagian) Malkasian, and young daughter, Irene (Zarouhi), to join him in America. Upon his wife's arrival, Sarkis, a carpenter by trade, built the first

Turkish-style bath house (hamam) in New England. With the success of the bath, the Malkasian family enjoyed some prosperity for the next few years.

Then World War I broke out in Europe, and with it, more than one-and-a-half million Armenian men, women, and children were killed in the first genocide of the 20th century. The entire Sahagian, Malkasian, and Mooradian clans of Pazmashen were lost.

Fortunately, my grandfather Eli, a young man by then, arrived in Whitinsville just before the massacres that wiped out his hometown. Five years later, he and my grandmother Irene, both born in a town that no longer existed and then living in Whitinsville, married. They bore three children (Warren, Anjel, and Arthur) and struggled through the Depression. Eli, like my great-grandfather Sarkis before him, worked in the Whitin Machine Works foundry. To help make ends meet, my grandmother sewed fancy hats in a sweatshop in Upton, Massachusetts.

Those were lean times. To eat, the family relied on vegetables my grandmother grew in a huge garden behind the house on Church Street and eggs laid by chickens my father kept in a coop. Breakfast consisted of bread and cheese or yogurt and an apple. Sunday dinner after church was the big family meal of the week. If they were lucky, maybe a chicken would be included.

Then in 1941, my family, like most immigrant families with sons, sent their boys to fight for the Allies in World War II. By the 1950s, my family had worked hard to fit in and become Americans. English, not Armenian, was spoken in the home, meat-stuffed vegetables had been supplanted by meat and potatoes on a plate, and two out of three of my grandparents' children, including my father, chose non-Armenian spouses. My family's Armenian identity was melting into the American pot.

Then in 1975, Alex Haley's message in *Roots* opened the door for all ethnic groups in the country to preserve and document their past.

This opening coincided with a decade of heavy Armenian immigration from the Middle East of people wanting to escape civil war in Beirut, Lebanon, and growing nationalist sentiments elsewhere. Among them were many members of my future husband's extended family. With them came hummus, baba ghanoush, and tabouli—delicious "little starter dishes" called mezze that they had assimilated into their kitchens from Arab neighbors.

Finally, in 1992, my husband and I honeymooned in Armenia—a republic reborn on the heels of the breakup of the Soviet Union.

Back in 1900, when my great-grandfather Sarkis arrived in America, no one cooked or ate meat off a skewer. Yet today, across the United States, restaurants serve pilaf and shish kebab, both signature Armenian dishes, as standard American fare. Sharing recipes and kitchen wisdom with neighbors and friends and family members is a universal passion of all cooks—everywhere.

By joining me in my newly discovered passion for the food of my ancestry, you too will be participating in the celebration of ethnicity that is taking place in all American kitchens today. I am honored to be a part of this celebration, and I believe that, no matter what national origin you claim, you will find yourself, and your own family's history, reflected in the simple elegance of the healthy dishes you will explore on these pages. It's time to come inside and discover the accessible yet still exotic Armenian table.

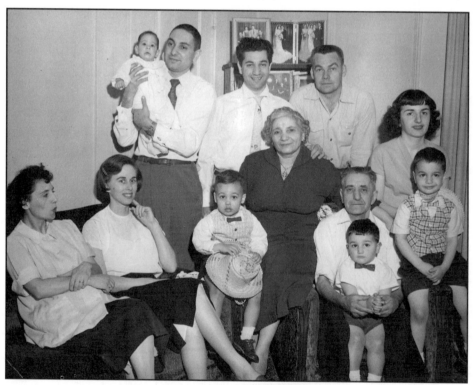

The Mooradian Family. Easter, 1956.
Whitinsville, Massachusetts.

APPETIZERS
&
SPREADS

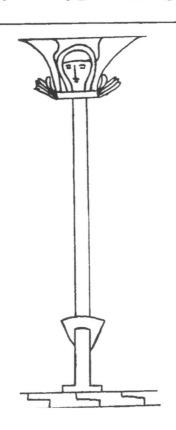

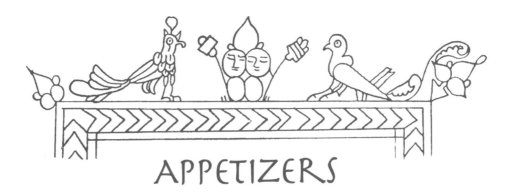

APPETIZERS

Rice-Stuffed Grape Leaves

Yalanchi Sarma

Makes 100

My stuffed grape leaves, called yalanchi in Turkish, are tarter and lighter-tasting than most recipes. The secret is to use slightly less olive oil and a lot more lemon juice.

My mother-in-law taught me to line the pot with carrot strips. Carrots add a subtle sweetness to the stuffed leaves, and once cooked, make a delicious bonus dish.

Serve stuffed grape leaves when entertaining large numbers of family and friends. They are also an important no-meat Lenten dish.

100 grape leaves, 4 bundles of small-sized leaves (page 28)
1¼ cups olive oil
¼ cup water
8 large onions, chopped
1½ cups short-grain white rice or medium-grain bulgur
2 bunches fresh flat-leaf parsley, finely chopped
2 teaspoons salt
2 tablespoons tomato paste
1 tablespoon sugar
1 teaspoon ground black pepper

2 - 3 tablespoons snipped fresh dill
2 tablespoons dried mint
Juice of 4 lemons
2 - 4 carrots, cut into long strips
2 - 3 lemons, cut in wedges
Fresh flat-leaf parsley sprigs

1. If using store-bought grape leaves, rinse them several times in water, draining each time. If using fresh or frozen grape leaves, plunge leaves in boiling salted water until the color darkens to olive, about 1 minute. Remove immediately, rinse with cold water, and drain.

2. Heat the olive oil and water in a large, deep-sided skillet. Add the onions and cook over medium-low heat until tender, about 30 minutes. Add the rice, parsley, and salt. Cover and simmer about 15 minutes.

3. Meanwhile, combine the tomato paste, sugar, black pepper, dill, 1 tablespoon dried mint, and juice from 3 of the lemons in a bowl. Stir into the rice, cover, and simmer another 10 minutes. Remove from heat.

4. Line the bottom of a large pot with grape leaves. Arrange the carrot strips lengthwise over the grape leaves across the bottom of the pot.

5. Taking one grape leaf at a time, trim the stem to a stub, if necessary. Place the leaf in the center of a small plate or work surface, vein side up, stem-end pointing down (towards you). Place a spoonful of rice stuffing into the center of the leaf. Fold the bottom up over the stuffing and the sides in toward the center and roll upward (away from you). Roll snugly. The rolled leaf will resemble a small hot dog.

6. As each leaf is rolled, arrange it in the pot on top of the carrot strips. After all the leaves are rolled, set a dinner plate, eating side down, on top of the pile of rolled grape leaves. This will secure them in place during cooking.

7. Bring 3 cups of water, the remaining mint, and the juice from the remaining lemon to a boil in a different pot. When boiling, pour the liquid into the pot holding the stuffed grape leaves. Cover, and bring the liquid quickly back to a boil over high heat. Lower the heat and simmer, covered, until the grape leaves are tender. This may take as little as 30 minutes if you used tender fresh leaves to as long as 1 hour if you used store-bought leaves, which can be thick and tough.

8. Remove from heat. Pour off excess water immediately. Let cool in the pot, still covered with the dinner plate, for at least 30 minutes before removing the stuffed leaves to a serving platter.

9. Garnish with cooked carrot strips, lemon wedges, and parsley. Cover with plastic wrap and refrigerate until serving. Traditionally, stuffed grape leaves are served slightly chilled or at room temperature as an appetizer. You can also serve them hot with a dollop of cool plain yogurt on top. This party-sized recipe yields enough to experiment.

❧ Fresh Grape Leaves ❧

3 hours of picking yields 300 to 325 leaves

Late spring is the time to gather and store fresh young grape leaves for the fall and winter, when Rice-Stuffed Grape Leaves (Yalanchi Sarma, page 25) and Lamb-Stuffed Grape Leaves (Sarma, page 160) are traditionally prepared and eaten. Depending on where you live and how quickly Mother Nature has warmed the earth, the perfect days to forage for wild grape leaves in New England will arrive as early as Memorial Day and last until the third week in June. Beyond that, the leaves become too tough to be appetizing.

Foraging for wild grape leaves was a necessity for my grandmother and her generation of cooks. Today, grape leaves pickled in jars of brine are available in most markets, but my guess is that once you've picked your own wild leaves, foraging will become an annual event for you, too.

Grape leaf picking requires some planning. Scout out vines with accessible leaves early. Wild grapes tend to grow along roadsides and on stone fences. Avoid pollution by choosing vines not growing near major roads. Once you've located your vines, set aside about six hours for this culinary adventure. Plan on three hours of picking followed by three hours of washing and bundling. It's a worthwhile investment.

Grape leaf picking is especially fun to do with a friend or your children. Warn your companions to wear long pants, socks, and sneakers, because poison ivy, insects, and spiders are notorious companions of wild grapes. Protective clothing is especially important in New England, where Lyme Disease-carrying deer ticks are common.

Once you've located some healthy, accessible vines, grab a few large paper bags and pick all the young light-green leaves that still have a shine to them. The best leaves are about 3-inches in diameter, but I harvest just about any leaf that is full-bodied, healthy, and tender. Use your thumbnail to cut off the stem as close to the bottom of the leaf as possible. Pick until your bags are filled or until you're satisfied or ready to go home. I start early in the morning with the goal of being home by lunchtime.

Back in your kitchen, fill the sink with cold water and float the leaves in the sink. If there are two of you, have one person wash the leaves while the other person trims, sorts for size, and bundles. The leaves may be covered with pollen, spider webs, or insects. So wash each leaf well, both front and back, under running tap water.

Set the clean leaves on the counter next to the sink. Trim the stems if necessary and sort the leaves by size. I usually have small-sized and large-sized piles. Once in piles, count out stacks of 25 leaves. Roll them, jelly-roll style, and tie each bundle with thin kitchen string. Place bundles in freezer bags and freeze. The leaves freeze really well.

My normal harvest usually results in 10 small-leaf bundles and 3 large-leaf bundles. One Rice-Stuffed Grape Leaves appetizer recipe (page 25) calls for four bundles, plus a bundle for lining the pan and extras. You should have enough grape leaves for two party-sized recipes and one dinner-sized Lamb-Stuffed Grape Leaves recipe (page 160).

When you're ready to use the leaves, bring a large pot of water to a boil, snip the bundling string, and plunge the frozen bundles into the boiling water. With a wooden spoon, gently poke at the bundles until the leaves unroll and darken to a deep green color. This should take about 5 minutes. Rinse immediately in cold water. Set leaves aside while you prepare the stuffing.

At the end of the day you'll be tired, but it will be a "good tired," the kind that is filled with pride about the work you've done. You might not want to see another grape leaf for a while, though. Our grandmothers may have felt the same. After spending a spring day harvesting wild leaves, it's little wonder that stuffing those leaves became an autumn culinary tradition!

Special Equipment:
String for bundling

Stuffed Mussels

Midya Dolma

Makes about 40

My grandmother didn't relax on the beach the way we did during summer days on the New England shore. She never changed into a bathing suit, and she wouldn't even consider swimming in the ocean! She'd sit all day on a lawn chair under the umbrella—unless there were mussel-covered rocks nearby. Then she'd take off her stockings, grab a bucket, hike up her paisley-print housedress, and forage the rocks for wild mussels.

Mussels are still almost free even when bought from the fish department of your local supermarket, and they are still delicious, especially when filled with my non-traditional orzo-based stuffing.

The Stuffing:
1 onion, finely chopped
⅓ cup olive oil
¼ cup chopped Toasted Pine Nuts (page 43)
⅔ cup uncooked orzo
2 tablespoons chopped fresh flat-leaf parsley
¼ teaspoon ground allspice
1 can (14½ ounces) peeled, diced tomatoes
1 cup water
1 teaspoon salt
¼ teaspoon ground black pepper

1 pound fresh live mussels
Salt
2 lemons, cut in wedges
Fresh flat-leaf parsley sprigs

1. In a large deep-sided skillet, cook the onions in the olive oil over moderate heat, stirring occasionally, until tender, about 10 minutes.

2. Add the nuts and sauté for 2 minutes before adding the orzo, parsley, allspice, tomato, water, salt, and pepper. Stir, cover, and simmer gently for 15 minutes.

3. Meanwhile, scrub the mussels well with a stiff brush. Then place them in warm salted water until they open, about 5 minutes. Being careful not to separate the shells completely, insert a knife in the opening between the mussel's two shells and slide it towards the mussel joint. This will sever the closing mechanism.

4. Place a generous teaspoon of filling into each mussel shell and close the shell as well as possible. Arrange the stuffed mussels in the bottom of a large pot, packing them as close together as possible, layering if necessary. Once they are tightly packed in the pot, place a dinner plate, eating side down, on top. This keeps the mussels in place and eliminates the need to tie them closed with kitchen string. Add 1 cup of boiling water to the pot. Cover and simmer gently for 30 minutes. Turn the heat off and allow the mussels to cool in the pan.

5. Arrange the cooled mussels on a serving platter. Garnish with lemon wedges and parsley. Serve chilled or at room temperature.

Feta Cheese-Topped Eggplant Rounds

Makes 12

Here's a totally vegetarian, pizza-style dish that many proclaim to be one of the best original recipes in the collection.

Non-stick cooking spray
1 large eggplant, peeled and sliced into ¼-inch-thick rounds
Salt
½ pound feta cheese, crumbled (about 1½ cups)
2 large eggs
½ teaspoon ground black pepper
½ green bell pepper, minced
1 tablespoon olive oil, plus ¼ cup for brushing
½ onion, minced
2 tomatoes, minced
¼ cup chopped fresh flat-leaf parsley
1 tablespoon fresh lemon juice

1. Preheat the oven to 400 degrees. Spray two baking sheets evenly with cooking spray. Set aside.
2. Soak the eggplant rounds in a large bowl of generously salted cold water for at least 15 minutes. Soaking the rounds eliminates any bitterness, inhibits oil absorption, and firms the rounds to better support the topping.
3. While the eggplant is soaking, mix together the feta, eggs, and black pepper in a large bowl and set aside.
4. Cook the green pepper in a skillet with 1 tablespoon olive oil over low heat until the pepper softens, about 10 minutes. Add the onion. Continue to cook, stirring occasionally, until onions are tender, another 10 minutes. Remove from heat, and combine with the feta mixture. Add the tomatoes, parsley, and lemon juice. Toss until the topping ingredients are mixed well.
5. Now it's time to remove the eggplant rounds from the water. Pat them dry with paper towels, brush the top and bottom of each slice with olive oil,

and arrange the oiled rounds on the prepared baking sheets. Spread a spoonful of feta mixture on top of each round until covered.

6. Bake for 25 minutes.
7. Serve warm as an appetizer or as a side, complementing any of the grilled lamb dishes.

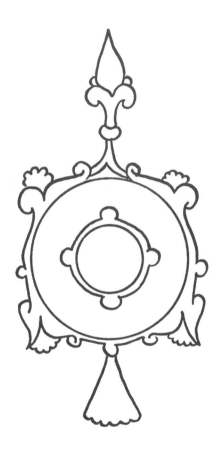

Syrian "Mortadella"

Makes 3 rolls

My mother-in-law taught me how to prepare this Syrian-influenced Armenian version of the popular Italian deli meat known by the same name. There are many variations, most of which call for hard-cooked egg in the center—with or without the pistachio nuts—but I think the egg makes it too heavy. The nuts add just enough color and flavor for me.

1 pound very lean (95% lean) ground beef or lamb (kheyma meat)
1 large egg
1 large egg, separated
1 small clove garlic, pressed
¼ teaspoon ground black pepper
¼ teaspoon ground allspice
½ teaspoon salt
⅓ cup plain bread crumbs
¼ cup shelled pistachio nuts (about 18 nuts, salted or unsalted)
¼ cup vegetable oil
2 tablespoons red wine vinegar

1. In a large mixing bowl, combine the meat with the whole egg and the egg yolk. Add the garlic, black pepper, allspice, and salt. Mix well before adding the bread crumbs. Knead the meat until the ingredients are evenly distributed throughout, then divide into 3 equal parts.
2. On a clean work surface, flatten and shape each section of meat into a circle about ⅛-inch thick. Place 6 pistachio nuts randomly on each circle. Roll up the circle, jelly-roll style, with the nuts inside. Mold the roll into a smooth-surfaced torpedo shape, wetting your hands with water if necessary.
3. Brush each roll with the reserved egg white. Heat the oil in a large skillet over moderately high heat until the oil is hot but not smoking. Fry each roll until well browned on all sides. Remove from heat. Drain excess oil off on paper towels.

4. Transfer the browned rolls to a large saucepan. Add the vinegar and enough water to cover the rolls. Cover the pot and quickly bring the liquid to a boil over high heat. Remove the cover, reduce the heat, and simmer until all of the liquid is evaporated, about 45 minutes.

5. Cool to room temperature before serving. Serve sliced with pita bread as an appetizer or bring this lunch meat along on your next picnic for a really special treat.

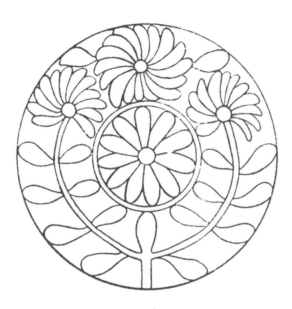

✑ Pickled Fresh Vegetables ҩ

Tourshi

The Armenian method of pickling fresh vegetables is quick, easy, and reliable. Raw or lightly poached vegetables are stored in glass jars and left to soak for about 10 days in a simple brine consisting of vinegar, salt, and water (see Note). The salt prevents bacterial growth by drawing moisture from the vegetables. The vegetables ferment in the brine and take on the taste of the other pickling ingredients. Use vegetables at their peak of freshness, and clean and wash them well before pickling. Regardless of the recipe, use perfectly clean glass jars with tightly fitting tops. Quart-sized mason jars with bands and dome lids work well. Sterilize jars and tops in boiling water for 10 minutes before use.

I've included four recipes for you to try. Pickled Carrots are my personal favorite, but the turnips and cauliflower and red cabbage will also please first-timers. Gourmets will want to try Pickled Eggplant.

My pickles are a tad spicy due to the sliver of hot pepper I add to every jar. Omit or cut the pepper portion in half, if desired. Serve as an appetizer, plain or with hummus. They are a titillating addition to almost any sandwich.

Brine

Makes 2 cups

1 tablespoon salt
1 cup water
1 cup white vinegar

1. Mix the brine in a clean glass or ceramic container. Dissolve the salt in the water and then stir in the vinegar. Completely cover the vegetables with this solution before tightly sealing the sterilized jar.

Pickled Carrots

Makes 4 quarts

3 pounds sliced carrots
3 cloves garlic, peeled and halved or quartered depending on size
3 - 4 whole peppercorns
1 - 2 sprigs fresh tarragon
Sliver serrano pepper, seeded
8 cups brine
4 (1-quart) jars

1. Pack the carrots in jars, alternating the garlic, peppercorns, and tarragon between them. Add the hot pepper slice.
2. Add enough brine to cover and seal the jar tightly.

Pickled Turnips

Makes 4 quarts

3 white turnips, peeled and quartered, then cut into
¼-inch thick slices
1 small beet, peeled and sliced
3 cloves garlic, peeled and halved or quartered depending on size
3 - 4 whole peppercorns
1 - 2 sprigs fresh tarragon
Sliver serrano pepper, seeded
8 cups brine
4 (1-quart) jars

1. Prepare according to the directions for Pickled Carrots above.

Pickled Cauliflower and Red Cabbage

Makes 4 quarts

1 white cauliflower, separated into flowerets
½ red cabbage, chunked
3 cloves garlic, peeled and halved or quartered depending on size
3 - 4 whole peppercorns
1 - 2 sprigs fresh tarragon
Sliver serrano pepper, seeded
8 cups brine
4 (1-quart) jars

1. Prepare according to the previous directions.

Pickled Eggplant

Makes 2 quarts

10 - 12 (5-inch to 6-inch long) finger eggplants
1 - 2 carrots, cut in slivers
3 cloves garlic, peeled and halved or quartered depending on size
1 bunch fresh flat-leaf parsley, chopped
4 cups brine
2 (1-quart) jars

1. Cut a small incision lengthwise in each eggplant.
2. Poach the eggplants in boiling water for 8 minutes until slightly softened. Remove from heat and drain well.
3. Stuff each eggplant with 2 carrot slivers, 4 garlic pieces, and parsley.
4. Arrange the stuffed eggplants in jars. Cover with brine and seal tightly.

Note: Store the jars in a temperate (55 to 60 degrees), dry place for about 10 days before opening. If possible, move the jars to an even cooler, drier place after those initial days. Once opened, these pickles must be refrigerated. They'll keep for up to a month in the refrigerator.

Armenian Meat Jerky

Soujouk

Makes 10 to 15 (1-pound) slabs

Soujouk is the Armenian version of beef jerky, only I prefer to make it with lamb. This recipe comes from Parouhi and Torkom Boyajian of Worcester, Massachusetts, and it's undoubtedly the best soujouk this side of the Atlantic.

Even into their 80s, the Boyajians kneaded their meat by hand—a feat befitting an entry in the *Guinness Book of Records*. I recommend using a tabletop mixer. If you don't have one, do what Armenian women throughout history have done: call a friend or relative who does have a mixer, double the batch, and work together. I often pair up with a culinary buddy anyway— because it's fun to chat and gossip during the two-day process that this recipe requires.

Wear your apron and roll up your sleeves, because making soujouk can be messy. This jerky is traditionally prepared in mid- to late autumn, after Indian summer but before the snow arrives, because before electricity and the use of fans, cooks depended upon the cool fall breezes to dry these heavily spiced, uncooked sausages. Be aware that during the weeks of drying you may drive the neighborhood dogs wild with the pungent smell of exotically spiced meat that will lace the crisp fall breeze.

15 - 18 pounds 80% lean ground lamb or beef (see Note)

The Spice Mix:
1½ cups ground cumin
¾ cup Hungarian hot paprika
¼ cup ground black pepper
⅛ cup cayenne
1½ tablespoons ground allspice
¾ cup salt

Special Equipment:
2 yards of unbleached muslin, washed without fabric softener
Needle and thread, or sewing machine, to sew bags
2 very large mixing bowls
Tabletop mixer with dough hook
Heavy rolling pin
String for hanging bags

1. A few days before you plan to prepare the meat, cut the washed muslin into 10 x 10-inch squares. Match 2 of the squares together and sew on 3 sides, leaving the top open. Sew as many bags as you can. Store the extra bags in a safe place, such as your linen closet, for use next year.

Day 1:

2. Allow the meat to come to room temperature while mixing the spices together in a medium-sized bowl.

3. In a very large mixing bowl, knead the spices into the meat with your hands until evenly distributed. Then, a few handfuls at a time, transfer the meat into the bowl of a tabletop mixer. Using a dough hook, blend at a low setting until the meat becomes smooth and pasty. Transfer the pasty meat into another very large bowl. Continue this process until all the meat has been mixed once with the dough hook.

4. Knead the meat again by hand, then mix all the meat again in the mixer, transferring it to a clean bowl. Cover with plastic wrap and let stand in the refrigerator for at least 8 hours (overnight).

Day 2:

5. The next day, mix the meat again thoroughly with the mixer, then roll the well-kneaded, pasty meat into balls the size of baseballs. Stuff each muslin bag with 3 to 4 balls. Finger the meat so that the balls blend together and fill the bag evenly.

6. Sew the top of each bag closed by hand. Then, with a rolling pin, roll each bag into a slab, about 1-inch thick. Work out any air bubbles. Poke two holes in the top of each bag and loop string through each hole, so the bag can be hung.

7. Hang each bag in a cool, dry, breezy place like a screened three-season porch, at about 50 degrees, until completely dry (about 4 weeks). I hang my bags on broomsticks hung between two lawn chairs or ladders in a clean, empty garage and place a fan set on low in front of the bags to promote air circulation during the days. Depending on the weather, I turn off the fan at night, because you do not want the meat to freeze. Every day or two, I turn the bags or move the fan so that the opposite side of the bags faces the fan-induced breeze. This helps to ensure even drying. The jerky is dry when it is very firm when squeezed. If you are not sure, make a 1-inch-deep cut into a slab. The dried jerky will be brown with a slightly pink center.

8. Once dry, peel off the muslin bag and discard. Wrap each slab in plastic wrap, covered with a layer of foil, and store in the freezer. Technically, soujouk will keep for eternity. In my family, we try to make 1 recipe last us until the following November. Be careful. There are many soujouk lovers out there who will be more than willing to raid your stash. Slice thin, serve sparingly, and enjoy! This jerky is especially tasty when served with an ice-cold beer.

Note: Beef is more commonly used than lamb. Some people even mix the two. I'm a purist so use one or the other.

☙ Toasted Pumpkin Seeds ❧

Makes about ½ cup

Toasted pumpkin seeds are a fall treat brimming with protein, low in fat, and high in fiber. Pan-frying slowly toasts the fresh seeds in their natural juice and helps retain the fresh squash flavor.

Fresh raw pumpkin seeds from 1 pumpkin (about ½ cup)
½ teaspoon olive oil
Dash of salt to taste

1. Remove the seeds from a fresh pumpkin. Place seeds in a strainer and rinse with cold water. Pick out any remaining pulp. Transfer the washed seeds to a paper towel and pat dry. Carve the pumpkin into a jack-o-lantern, or try the Fresh Candied-Pumpkin Slices (page 256).
2. Cook the seeds in a heavy-bottomed skillet over moderate heat, stirring constantly, until the seeds puff and turn golden, about 15 minutes. Remove from heat and cool the seeds on a paper towel.
3. Transfer the cooled seeds to a serving bowl. Stir in oil and lightly salt to taste. Eat immediately or store in an airtight container.

Note: This recipe works well with squash seeds, too.

✑ Toasted Pine Nuts ✑

Makes 1 cup

Toasting brings out the rich flavor and makes this nut easier to digest.

1 cup raw pine nuts

1. In a large heavy-bottomed skillet, sauté nuts over medium heat, stirring frequently, until golden brown. Remove from heat and cool on a paper towel.
2. Use immediately or transfer to an airtight container and freeze for later.

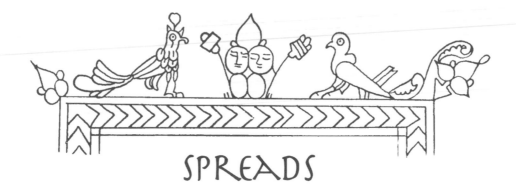

SPREADS

❧ Chickpeas with Tahini ❧

Hummus

Serves 10

Best known by its Arabic name, hummus is the most famous of the Middle Eastern dips. People rave about my husband's hummus. So much so that "Vatche's Hummus" is a required dish at family gatherings. My husband shared his secrets to preparing great hummus with me, and now I'll share them with you.

Secret number 1:   Do not add garlic! I know many people put garlic in their hummus as a matter of routine, but I oppose doing so because even a little garlic overpowers the gentle blend of flavors that characterize this spread, and the dish quickly becomes all about the garlic. Follow this recipe exactly and I guarantee your hummus will be the hit of the party.

Secret number 2:   A tiny bit of sugar improves the taste dramatically.

Secret number 3:   Delicious hummus can start with "ready-to-serve" chickpea dip from a can, so you do not have to begin the preparation process from scratch if you don't want to. Instead, open a can of already prepared chickpea dip made in Lebanon and sold here in Middle Eastern stores. Then doctor it with additional tahini and lemon juice according to the second set of instructions on the next page.

From Scratch:
2 cans (15½ ounces) chickpeas, drained, rinsed, and mashed
⅓ cup water
Juice of 2 large lemons
4 tablespoons well-stirred tahini
1 teaspoon salt
½ teaspoon ground cumin
½ teaspoon sugar

Special Equipment:
Food processor

1. In the bowl of a food processor, combine the mashed chickpeas, water, lemon juice, tahini, salt, cumin, and sugar. Process into a smooth paste.
2. Hummus should have the consistency of a loose paste that is easy to dip or spread; add water or lemon juice to thin it if necessary.
3. Once the consistency is right, spoon into a shallow serving dish. Serve with sliced pita bread or chips.

From a Can:
2 - 3 tablespoons well-stirred tahini
1½ tablespoons water
Juice of 1 large lemon
½ teaspoon ground cumin
1 can (13¼ ounces) chickpea dip (see Note)

1. Combine the tahini, water, and lemon juice in a bowl. Whip into a paste. Stir in cumin.
2. Add the chickpea dip. Mix to a smooth paste; adjust to taste. I don't usually add sugar because the prepared paste tends to be a sweeter anyway.

Note: We found Cortas brand to be the best for both taste and consistency.

☙ Eggplant with Tahini ❧

Baba Ghanoush

Serves 6

Pull the grill out of the shed, stoke up the coals, and roast an eggplant whole. It's that easy to prepare this popular Middle Eastern spread that was first introduced into American Armenian cuisine in the late 1970s when many Lebanese Armenians fled to the United States to escape the civil war that was ravaging that tiny, cosmopolitan country.

1 medium-sized eggplant
1 clove garlic, pressed
¼ cup well-stirred tahini
2 tablespoons extra-virgin olive oil
¼ teaspoon salt
½ teaspoon ground cumin
½ teaspoon cayenne, plus an extra shake to garnish
Juice of 1 lemon
Fresh flat-leaf parsley

Special Equipment:
Food processor (optional)

1. Place the whole eggplant directly on the grill over medium-hot coals and roast until the skin is charred—the eggplant will become soft and collapse like a deflated balloon. Remove from heat and let cool.
2. Peel and turn the pulp into the bowl of a food processor or a medium-sized mixing bowl.
3. Add all of the remaining ingredients and blend into a loose, smooth paste, about 2 minutes. An electric mixer or manual masher may also be used but reducing the pulp to a smooth paste may take longer.
4. Turn the spread into a shallow serving dish. Garnish with an extra shake of cayenne and parsley. Serve at room temperature with fresh pita slices or Toasted Pita Chips (page 191).

Note: Rather than starting from scratch, spoon 1 can (12 ounces) prepared baba ghanoush—my preference is Cortas brand—into a mixing bowl. Stir in 1 tablespoon tahini, ⅛ teaspoon ground cumin, a pinch of cayenne, and the juice of 1 lemon. Adjust to taste. This version is just as good, if not better, than the first and no one will know the difference. Smile and accept your guests' compliments without guilt.

☙ Zesty White Bean Dip ❧

Serves 8

This spread offers a wonderful alternative to hummus or baba ghanoush. Today, especially in our health-conscious world, white kidney beans are popular legumes. I have paired the smooth-tasting beans with hot peppers and the traditional lemon–olive oil dressing of the Armenian kitchen to make a delicious dip with a tantalizing kick.

2 cans (14 ounces) white kidney beans, rinsed and drained
1 small clove garlic
¾ teaspoon salt
¼ teaspoon ground black pepper
¼ teaspoon cayenne, plus a dash to garnish
Juice of 1 lemon
4 - 5 drops Tabasco sauce
¼ cup extra-virgin olive oil

Special Equipment:
Food processor (optional)
Mortar and pestle

1. Place the beans in a large mixing bowl and mash to a paste with a hand-held potato masher or fork. Or put the beans in the bowl of a food processor and blend until smooth.
2. Using a mortar and pestle, crush the garlic clove with the salt into a paste; add to the beans. Sprinkle the black pepper and cayenne evenly over the top. Stir well to combine.
3. In a second bowl, combine the lemon juice, Tabasco, and olive oil. Whisk before adding to the white bean paste. Stir, mash, or pulse until the spread is smooth and creamy.
4. Transfer to a serving dish and top with a sprinkle of cayenne. Serve this dip slightly chilled or at room temperature with fresh pita, Toasted Pita Chips (page 191), or a slice of home-baked Savory Dill Bread (page 201).

Note: If you don't have a food processor, don't despair; the dip tastes the same when made by hand, but the final texture is a little lumpier.

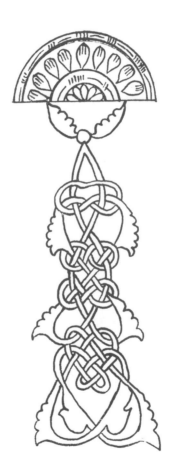

Hummus with Tangy Yogurt Sauce

Fatté

Serves 6

Called fatté in Arabic, this elaboration on basic hummus is the Middle Eastern version of nachos.

Chickpeas with Tahini (Hummus, page 44)
Toasted Pita Chips (page 191)

The Topping:
5 tablespoons Yogurt Cheese (Labni, page 229)
¼ cup water
2 tablespoons butter, melted
Dash of ground sumac (see Note)
Sprinkle of cayenne

1. Spread one batch of hummus in a large shallow serving dish. Arrange tortilla chip-sized pieces of Toasted Pita Chips on top.
2. Prepare the topping by mixing the yogurt cheese and water together in a small bowl. First, drizzle the thinned yogurt cheese over the pita chips, then drizzle the melted butter on top.
3. Finally, garnish with sumac and cayenne to taste.

Note: Sumac is made from the berries of a wild bush that grows throughout the Mediterranean. It is burgundy or rust-colored and has a tangy, lemony taste. It is most often sprinkled on top of food as a condiment. Unfortunately, it has no good substitute, so if you can't find it, just omit it.

ᥲ Spicy Hot Walnut Spread ᥱ

Muhammarah

Serves 6

Known in Arabic as muhammarah, this spread is "taste bud dynamite!" It's guaranteed to spice up the party as well as the appetite.

1 tablespoon cayenne or Hungarian hot paprika
1 teaspoon water
1 cup plain bread crumbs
½ cup water
1 cup coarsely chopped walnuts
1 tablespoon sugar
½ teaspoon salt
2 tablespoons pomegranate molasses or concentrated juice
⅓ cup olive oil
Juice of ½ lemon
Fresh chopped flat-leaf parsley

1. In a small bowl, mix the cayenne and water together. Set aside.
2. In a larger mixing bowl, combine the bread crumbs, water, walnuts, sugar, salt, pomegranate molasses, and olive oil.
3. Add the lemon juice and cayenne water. Mix well.
4. Spoon the thick and chunky spread into a shallow serving dish, garnish with parsley, and serve with a generous portion of pita slices.

✑ Carrot-Potato Dip ✑
with Marinated Artichoke Hearts

Serves 12

Beautifully festive, easy to make, and full of spicy flavor, this starter dish is my own creation. Even the toughest-to-please guests will express their delight over the smooth, gently spiced orange center surrounded by a zesty wheel of green artichokes.

The Dip:
1¼ pounds (8 to 9) carrots, peeled and sliced into thin rounds
1 small garlic clove, minced
1 pound (3 medium-sized) potatoes, peeled and sliced thin
1½ teaspoons salt
2 teaspoons ground cumin
3 tablespoons olive oil
2 tablespoons red wine vinegar
Large pinch of cayenne

The Artichokes (see Note):
2 cans (12 - 14 ounces) artichoke hearts
½ cup extra-virgin olive oil
¼ cup balsamic vinegar
½ teaspoon dry mustard
½ teaspoon salt
¼ teaspoon ground black pepper
Fresh flat-leaf parsley sprigs

Special Equipment:
Food processor (optional)

1. Combine the carrots and garlic in a pot. Put the potatoes into a separate pot. Add enough water to cover each. Bring both to a boil over high heat.

2. Lower the heat under both pots, cover, and simmer until soft, about 20 minutes or until a fork slides into the potato and carrot pieces easily.

3. Remove from heat and drain each pot. Transfer the carrots, garlic, and potatoes to the bowl of a food processor or a large mixing bowl.

4. Add the salt, cumin, oil, vinegar, and cayenne. Blend until smooth. If you don't have a food processor, whip the ingredients with an electric mixer or mash with a hand-held potato masher until the spread is a smooth and creamy paste.

5. To prepare the artichoke hearts, drain and cut the hearts into bite-sized pieces. Place in a mixing bowl and set aside.

6. In a small mixing bowl, whisk the oil, balsamic vinegar, dry mustard, salt, and black pepper together until blended. Pour over the artichoke pieces and toss to cover.

7. Scoop the dip into the middle of a large serving plate. Surround the pretty orange-colored spread with artichokes. Garnish the center with a few sprigs of parsley.

8. Best served at room temperature with a generous portion of Toasted Pita Chips (page 191).

Note: Substitute your favorite brand of marinated artichoke hearts if you don't have the time or inclination to prepare them yourself.

Spiced Feta Cheese Spread

Shenglish

Serves 8

½ pound feta cheese (preferably French), crumbled (about 1½ cups)
1 teaspoon ground cumin
½ teaspoon dried thyme
½ teaspoon dried oregano
½ teaspoon cayenne
1 teaspoon chopped fresh mint, or ¼ teaspoon dried mint
2 tablespoons extra-virgin olive oil

1. Put the feta in a bowl. Add the remaining ingredients and mash with a fork until spices are spread uniformly throughout the cheese.
2. Spread in a shallow serving dish and serve at room temperature with pita slices, Toasted Pita Chips (page 191), or Armenian Cracker Bread (page 189) on the side. Yum! Yum!

❧ Kalamata Olive Spread ❧

Serves 6

The Armenian kitchen is not complete without olives. This spread has been christened "fabulous" by numerous olive lovers. Offer it as an appetizing prelude to grilled lamb and tip the scales of human emotion in your favor.

2 cups whole kalamata black olives, pitted
1 small onion, finely chopped
⅓ cup finely chopped fresh flat-leaf parsley
⅓ cup coarsely chopped walnuts
Juice of 1 lemon
⅓ cup tomato paste
½ teaspoon cayenne
½ teaspoon ground cumin
½ teaspoon salt
Fresh flat-leaf parsley sprigs

1. Rinse the olives well under cold water. Transfer them to a large bowl and soak in a generous amount of cold water for at least 2 hours; change the water once about halfway through the soaking time.
2. Drain the soaked olives. Cut each into 4 to 6 pieces and place in a mixing bowl. Stir in the onion, parsley, and walnuts.
3. In a separate bowl, combine the lemon juice, tomato paste, cayenne, cumin, and salt. Pour over the olives and mix until well combined.
4. Spread on a serving plate. Garnish with parsley and serve at room temperature with pita slices or crackers.

Black Olive and Yogurt Cheese Spread

Serves 6

September begins "Potluck Season." From September until the end of June, notices from school, church, and professional groups pour in with invitations to potluck get-togethers. Quickly, I find myself short on time and long on commitments. For those of you in similar situations, try this make-ahead spread—its flavors blend and become better after a day or so in the refrigerator.

1 cup Yogurt Cheese (Labni, page 229)
¼ cup black pitted olives
1 small garlic clove, pressed
1 tablespoon chopped fresh mint, or 1 teaspoon dried mint
1 tablespoon snipped fresh dill, or 1 teaspoon dried dill
¼ teaspoon salt
Fresh mint

1. Make the yogurt cheese or substitute labni. Keep refrigerated.
2. Rinse the olives well under cold water, then place in a bowl and soak in a generous amount of cold water for 1 to 2 hours; change the water halfway through the soaking time. Drain and coarsely chop, then set aside.
3. In a small mixing bowl, combine the garlic, mint, and dill. Fold into the yogurt cheese. Gently stir in the chopped olives, and salt to taste.
4. Best if covered and refrigerated for at least a few hours before serving. Garnish with fresh mint and serve with pita slices or crackers.

FIRST
COURSES

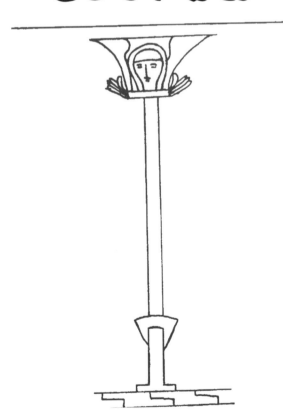

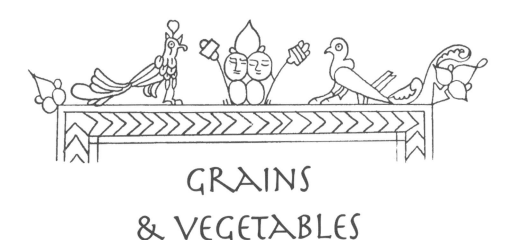

GRAINS & VEGETABLES

Bulgur Pilaf

Serves 4

The Hittites were among the first people to cultivate wheat. Armenians are direct descendents of the Hittites, who tilled the hills and mountains of Anatolia and the Caucasus from as early as 3000 BC, and many Hittite-derived words are still in use in modern-day Armenian. Now, that's ancient!

Bulgur, also known as cracked wheat, was originally developed as a preservation method in which the whole-wheat kernels were boiled outdoors in huge cauldrons and then dried in the sun. This was always done in very hot weather so that the wheat dried completely in one day. If left overnight, it tended to mildew. The sun not only dried the wheat, but also preserved it. Since ancient times, people have known that wheat is the only cereal that, if dried properly, becomes absolutely resistant to bugs or mold and can be kept for years. Think of bulgur as a permanent pantry.

Many conquerors in history—Mongols, Persians, Turks—trudged through the Armenian homeland. Most would have starved had it not been for the huge stores of cracked wheat they found in the homes and villages of historic Armenia.

Essentially, bulgur is to the Armenian kitchen what pasta is to the Italian. It's a staple—rich in nutrition, fiber, and history.

The key to great pilaf is to make one batch at a time and to resist stirring it again after the first "big stir" you give it just after adding the grain to the boiling chicken broth.

1 nest fine curly vermicelli
1 tablespoon butter
1 cup coarse-grain bulgur
1½ cups chicken broth (see Note)

1. Break the vermicelli nest into small pieces with your hands into a small (1-quart) saucepan. Add the butter. Over low heat, stirring constantly, cook the vermicelli until just golden. Once it begins to brown it will brown quickly, so be careful not to burn it. Remove from heat.
2. In a separate saucepan, bring the broth to a boil.
3. Pour the boiling broth into the saucepan with the browned vermicelli. Add the bulgur, and give the pot one big stir. Cover and simmer over moderate to low heat until the broth is absorbed, about 14 minutes.
4. Let stand, covered, 5 minutes before serving.

Note: For most American-born Armenian cooks there is no substitute brand for College Inn. Use 1 (14½ ounces) can.

Rice Pilaf

Serves 4

The rice has to be Uncle Ben's, and the chicken broth has to be College Inn, no substitutes allowed, if you want to re-create the taste and texture of the rice pilaf so many American-born Armenians were weaned on.

1 nest fine curly vermicelli
1 tablespoon butter
1½ cups chicken broth
1 cup long-grain white rice

1. Break the vermicelli nest into small pieces with your hands into a small (1-quart) saucepan. Add the butter. Over low heat, stirring constantly, cook the vermicelli until just golden. Once it begins to brown it will brown quickly, so be careful not to burn it. Remove from heat.
2. In a separate saucepan, bring the broth to a boil.
3. Pour the boiling broth into the saucepan with the browned vermicelli. Add the rice, and give the pot one big stir. Cover and simmer over moderate to low heat until the broth is absorbed, about 14 minutes.
4. Let stand, covered, 5 minutes before serving.

Rice Pilaf
with Pomegranate and Toasted Pine Nuts

Serves 4

The exotic pomegranate is an ancient fruit some claim dates back to the Garden of Eden. Its juicy, bright-red seeds add symbolism and tangy flavor to this special pilaf.

Rice Pilaf, prepared according to the instructions on page 61
1 pomegranate (see Note)
¼ cup Toasted Pine Nuts (page 43)

1. Begin by preparing the rice pilaf.
2. While the pilaf is cooking, remove the seeds from the pomegranate; discard peel and membrane. Set aside.
3. Once the liquid has completely absorbed into the rice (after Step 3, page 61), stir in the pomegranate seeds and pine nuts and let stand, covered, for 5 minutes.
4. Turn into a large pretty dish and serve warm.

Note: Buy the reddest pomegranate you can find. The ruby red juice of this fruit is pretty, but the stains it can leave on your clothes are not. To prevent unwanted squirting, immerse the fruit in a large bowl of water set in the sink and separate the seeds underwater. Drain before using.

✑ Green Beans in Tomato Sauce ✑

Fasoulia

Serves 6

This dish may sound a bit bland to some, but my family loves the clean taste fresh green beans offer when accented with tomato and olive oil. For those of you who want to jazz it up, add some chopped onion or try it with lamb stew meat as suggested in the recipe that follows.

1½ pounds green beans, tips removed and cut into 1-inch lengths
⅓ cup tomato paste
¼ cup olive oil
1 teaspoon salt
½ teaspoon ground black pepper

1. Put the beans in a medium-sized (2-quart) saucepan and cover with water, about 4 cups. Stir in tomato paste, olive oil, salt, and pepper.
2. Cover and bring to a boil. Lower heat and simmer, covered, until very tender, about 25 minutes. In the time-honored tradition of Armenian cooks, green beans are considered more delicious when well cooked. When cooked slowly, these beans are soft and buttery.
3. Serve with pilaf.

Lamb and Green Beans

Serves 6

1 pound lamb stew meat
1 medium onion, diced
1 tablespoon olive oil
Green Beans in Tomato Sauce, prepared as described on page 63

1. Brown the stew meat on all sides in a large deep-sided skillet over medium-high heat. When the meat is browned, add enough water to the pan to cover about ¾ of the meat. Lower heat, cover, and simmer for 1 hour, until meat is cooked through and tender. Remove from heat and cool to room temperature. (I often stop here, cover the pan, and put it in the refrigerator until the next day.)
2. Once cooled, cut the meat from the bones, eliminating fatty sections. Put the meat chunks in a medium-sized saucepan. Transfer at least ¼ cup of jelled juices from the pan to the saucepan. (If you stopped and put the meat in the refrigerator as suggested in Step 1, skim off the fat that has solidified on top, but keep the juices, which add a lot of flavor!)
3. Sauté the onion and oil in a skillet over medium heat until the onion is soft and golden. Transfer to the saucepan.
4. Finish this dish by following the directions for Green Beans in Tomato Sauce (page 63).

❧ Cumin-Glazed Carrots ❧

Serves 4

1 pound baby carrots (about 3 cups)
2 tablespoons olive oil
¼ teaspoon ground cumin
1 cup water
Juice of 1 lemon
1 teaspoon honey
½ teaspoon salt
¼ teaspoon ground black pepper

1. Cook the carrots with the oil and cumin in a heavy-bottomed saucepan over moderate heat, stirring, until well coated, about 1 minute.
2. Add the remaining ingredients and simmer, uncovered, stirring occasionally, until the liquid is evaporated and the carrots are tender and glazed, about 20 minutes.
3. Serve warm, at room temperature, or chilled as a snack.

✍ Vegetable Medley ✍

Turlu

Serves 8

This dish has endless variations, depending on the season and the vegetables that are in your refrigerator or on sale at the market. Turlu is often made when it's time to use aging vegetables. Many recipes call for throwing whatever you have, or want to get rid of, into a baking pan and roasting until slightly charred, but every time I tried that, the result was unappetizing. Finally, I discovered that adding olive oil and a little sugar made all the difference.

8 finger eggplants
Salt
2 medium onions, cut lengthwise into ¼-inch-thick wedges
6 tablespoons olive oil
1 tomato, coarsely chopped, plus 1½ cups drained chopped tomatoes
(reserved from Stuffed Tomatoes recipe, page 94), or substitute
1 can (14¼ ounces) peeled, diced tomatoes
1 large bunch fresh flat-leaf parsley, chopped
2 tablespoons chopped fresh basil
Juice of 2 lemons
2 tablespoons plus 1 tablespoon sugar
1 teaspoon salt
½ cup water

1. Preheat the oven to 400 degrees.
2. Halve eggplants lengthwise and score flesh ½-inch deep in a crosshatch pattern to make 1-inch squares (do not cut through the skin). Arrange eggplant halves, side by side, cut sides up, on a baking sheet and season with salt. Bake until softened, about 15 minutes. Remove from the oven and transfer to a roasting pan just large enough to fit the eggplant fingers in one layer.
3. Cook the onions in 3 tablespoons olive oil in a large deep-sided skillet over moderate heat, stirring occasionally, until softened, about 10 minutes.

Remove skillet from heat and stir in the tomato, parsley, basil, lemon juice, 2 tablespoons sugar, and salt.

4. Pour over the softened eggplant.

5. In a separate bowl, combine the water, the remaining 3 tablespoons oil, and the remaining 1 tablespoon sugar. Stir until the sugar is completely dissolved, then add to the roasting pan. Cover the pan tightly with foil or a lid and bake for 45 minutes. Uncover and bake until the cooking liquid is reduced and the vegetables begin to caramelize, about another 30 minutes.

6. Serve hot as a complement to any of the meat dishes offered in this collection, alongside bulgur pilaf. Leftovers are fantastic served at room temperature the next day as a salad with pita or any of the Armenian flat breads.

Note: This dish may be made a day ahead. Cool completely before covering and chilling. The next day, bring the dish to room temperature before reheating, uncovered, until hot throughout, about 30 minutes.

Fried Eggplant with Yogurt Sauce

Serves 4

1 medium eggplant, peeled and sliced into ¼-inch-thick rounds
Salt
½ cup plain bread crumbs
2 - 3 large eggs, beaten until frothy
4 tablespoons (½ stick) butter
¼ cup olive oil

1 cup Yogurt Sauce (page 226)

1. Soak the eggplant rounds in a large bowl filled with cold, heavily salted water for at least 15 to 20 minutes. Remove the slices from the water and pat dry with a paper towel. Soaking the eggplant helps keep its shape when frying.
2. Place the bread crumbs in a shallow wide-mouth dish on a work space near the stove. Place the eggs in a similar dish next to it.
3. In a medium-sized skillet, heat the butter and olive oil over moderate heat.
4. In assembly-line fashion, taking 1 eggplant slice at a time, coat it with bread crumbs, then dip it in egg, so that both sides are coated. (Recipes you may be familiar with ask you to do the reverse, dip in egg first then in bread crumbs. Although counterintuitive, your fried eggplant will be tastier prepared my way.)
5. Drain off excess egg, then fry each round until golden brown on both sides in the prepared skillet. Drain on paper towels.
6. Serve hot or at room temperature piled on a serving platter with Yogurt Sauce as an accompaniment.

Note: Eggplant can be fried a day before serving and then refrigerated. Reheat in a low-temperature oven and serve.

❧ Grilled Eggplant ❧

Serves 8

This is an easy-to-make extra dish that complements any grilled meal.

1 large eggplant, cut into ¼-inch-thick rounds
⅓ cup olive oil or more to taste

1. Brush each eggplant round on both sides with olive oil.
2. Prepare a gas or charcoal grill. Grill the rounds directly on a lightly oiled grill rack, over moderately high heat, until browned, about 7 minutes per side. For extra-rich flavor, continue to brush the rounds with olive oil as they cook.
3. Remove from heat directly to a serving platter.

☙ Roasted Italian Peppers ❧

Serves 8

4 large Italian peppers
1 tablespoon olive oil (optional)
1 clove garlic, chopped (optional)

1. Prepare a gas or charcoal grill. Place the whole peppers directly on the grill rack over moderate heat. Grill, turning occasionally, until skins blister and blacken and the peppers soften and collapse, about 10 minutes.
2. Remove from heat and set aside to cool, about 15 minutes. (You can enclose the peppers in a bag while cooling so that they sweat and the skins slip off more easily, but I've never found the extra step made enough of a difference to warrant doing it.)
3. Peel skin. Remove stem and seeds. Then slice or pull into strips.
4. Serve as is or add olive oil and garlic.

Note: When stored in an airtight container, these peppers will keep for a few days in the refrigerator. For a real treat, try a slice of roasted pepper on your favorite sandwich.

☙ Brown Lentils and Rice ❧

Mujaddarah

Serves 8

Mujaddarah is an Arab dish that the Armenians have co-opted because it fits so well in their diet, especially during Lent. The Lenten fast practiced by the Armenian Orthodox Church eliminates all animal-derived products, including dairy, from the table. At first, adhering to the stiff ingredient guidelines of Lent may seem a near impossible task, requiring a great deal of self-discipline. But the traditional cuisine of the Armenian kitchen tailors itself effortlessly to the celebration of this time. Mujaddarah is a perfect addition to the Lenten table, and it's a healthy diversion at any time of the year.

The key to making great mujaddarah lies in the preparation of the onion. Slice the onion very, very thin and evenly, so that it browns uniformly in the olive oil until crispy but not burned.

1 cup brown lentils, picked clean of debris and rinsed, soaked in cold water for at least 1 hour, then rinsed again and drained
3 cups water
1 teaspoon salt
1 cup short-grain white rice or coarse-grain bulgur
1 medium onion, thinly sliced into ringlets
¼ cup olive oil

1. Add the water and salt to the soaked lentils and bring to a boil over high heat. Lower heat and simmer, covered, for 15 minutes. Add rice. Continue cooking, covered, for another 15 to 20 minutes, until the water is completely absorbed. Remove from heat and set aside.
2. In a small skillet, fry the onion in olive oil, over medium heat, until the onion slices are browned but not burned. Using a large slotted spoon, remove the onions from the skillet and drain them on paper towels. Once cooled, toss the crispy onions into the lentils.
3. Serve hot, at room temperature, or chilled. Great accompanied by a tossed green salad.

✑ Red Lentil Patties ✑

Vospov Kufteh

Serves 4

After more than 1700 years of Christianity, it's hard to separate anything the Armenians do from their religion, including what they eat. There are 180 fasting days in the religious calendar of the Armenian Apostolic Church. That's five days shy of half the year!

In ancient times, the faithful were asked to abstain from eating, but over the centuries, "doing with light sustenance" came to be known as fasting. Currently, the church has placed the limits at vegetable products, with the exception of honey, which is an animal product. Dairy (eggs, butter, cheese, milk, etc.) is also excluded. Some authorities allow the consumption of free-swimming species of fish, but not shellfish. Now you know why dishes based on lentils, beans, and chickpeas constitute a large number of traditional Armenian dishes!

Today, few faithful Armenians living in the United States regulate their diets according to the church calendar, but many continue to observe the Lenten fast. Vospov kufteh is the most famous of the Armenian Lenten dishes—the ingredients and their preparation respect the strictest interpretation of the church's dietary requirements, but the dish's full-bodied taste defies the concept of sacrifice. No matter what your culinary tendencies might be, this dish is a particularly good one to pull out of your chef's hat year-round.

1 cup red lentils, picked clean of debris and rinsed
3 cups water
½ cup fine-grain bulgur
1 teaspoon salt
1½ teaspoon ground cumin
2 medium onions, finely chopped and divided
½ teaspoon cayenne
1 tablespoon olive oil
1 small bunch fresh flat-leaf parsley, chopped

1. Place the lentils and water in a saucepan. Cover and bring to a boil. Lower heat and simmer, still covered, 10 to 15 minutes, until the lentils are tender. Red lentils cook quickly!
2. Add the bulgur, salt, and cumin. Stir well and turn off the heat.
3. In a skillet, sauté half the onion with the cayenne in the olive oil until the onion is translucent, about 10 minutes.
4. Combine onion with the lentil mixture. Let stand, uncovered, until cool, about 30 minutes.
5. Shape lentil mixture into egg-sized pieces or patties and arrange on a serving tray. Pile patties high with parsley and the remaining onion.
6. Serve at room temperature or chilled with a tossed green salad and pita or Armenian Cracker Bread (page 189).

☙ Potato-Onion Kibbeh ❧

Serves 8

Kibbeh is the Arabic word for a layered, one-pan dish. Serve this hearty and satisfying vegetarian kibbeh with any of my savory meat or poultry dishes.

4 large potatoes, peeled and cut in ¼-inch-thick slices
Salt
1 cup fine-grain bulgur, soaked
1 large onion, grated
½ cup finely chopped fresh flat-leaf parsley
1 teaspoon dried mint
½ teaspoon ground cumin
2 teaspoons salt
½ teaspoon ground black pepper
1 medium onion, sliced
½ cup olive oil

Special Equipment:
1 (9-inch square) baking pan

1. Place the potatoes in a large pot, cover with water, add salt, and boil until the potatoes are tender, about 25 minutes. Drain and mash. Set aside.
2. Place the bulgur in a medium-sized bowl. Add enough cold water to just cover the grain, stir, and let soak for 15 minutes. The bulgur will absorb the water and puff up.
3. Preheat the oven to 400 degrees.
4. In a large mixing bowl, combine the potatoes, soaked bulgur, grated onion, parsley, mint, cumin, salt, and pepper. Knead, moistening your hands occasionally with cold water, if necessary, until evenly combined.
5. Spread the sliced onion and ¼ cup olive oil on the bottom of the baking dish. Pat the potato mixture evenly over the raw onion slices. Pour the remaining ¼ cup oil evenly over the top and bake for 35 minutes or until golden brown on top.
6. Serve warm with a salad for a complete meatless meal.

Potato-Spinach Kibbeh

Serves 8

3 baking potatoes, peeled and cut into ¼-inch-thick slices
Salt
½ cup plain yogurt
1½ tablespoons butter
¼ teaspoon cayenne
1 large egg, beaten
½ pound feta cheese, crumbled (about 1½ cups)
10 ounces fresh spinach (about 8 cups), washed and chopped, or
1 package (10 ounces) frozen chopped spinach, thawed and drained
Dash of cayenne

Special Equipment:
1 (9-inch square) baking dish

1. Put the potatoes in a large pot. Add enough water to cover, salt generously, and bring to a boil over high heat. Lower heat and cook until the potatoes are tender, about 25 minutes. Drain, transfer to a large mixing bowl, and mash. (While you can prepare this recipe by hand, for best results whip the potatoes with an electric mixer on low until fluffy.)
2. Add the yogurt, butter, and cayenne; beat until just combined.
3. Add the egg. Beat until fluffy, about 1 minute. Fold in half of the crumbled feta cheese.
4. Preheat the oven to 425 degrees.
5. In a large skillet, bring ¼ cup water to a boil; add spinach. Toss for about 2 minutes until the fresh spinach wilts or the frozen spinach is slightly cooked. Drain, pressing out excess liquid, and coarsely chop, if necessary.
6. In a separate bowl, mix the remaining cheese with the spinach.
7. Assemble the layers by spreading half of the potato mixture into the baking dish, layering the spinach evenly on top, patting the remaining potato mixture over the spinach, and sprinkling the top with cayenne.
8. Bake, uncovered, for 15 minutes or until the top is lightly browned.
9. Serve hot with the main course of your choice.

Spinach Casserole

Serves 8

This scrumptious casserole is a stand-alone, meat-free comfort meal.

1 cup red lentils, picked clean of debris and rinsed
1 teaspoon ground cumin
½ teaspoon cayenne
1 bouillon cube, chicken or vegetable
1 cup coarse-grain bulgur
1 small clove garlic, finely chopped
1 medium onion, finely chopped
3 tablespoons olive oil
10 ounces fresh spinach (about 8 cups), washed and chopped
¼ cup chopped fresh flat-leaf parsley
½ pound feta cheese, crumbled (about 1½ cups)
3 large eggs, beaten
¼ cup balsamic vinegar
1 teaspoon salt
½ teaspoon ground black pepper
1 tomato, thinly sliced

1. Preheat the oven to 400 degrees. Lightly grease a medium- to large-sized casserole dish with olive oil.
2. Place the lentils in a small saucepan. Add 1½ cups water, cover, and bring to a boil. Skim off any froth that may accumulate on the surface as the lentils cook. Partially cover the saucepan by off-setting the cover so it leaves a generous crack, lower heat, and simmer for 15 minutes, or until all of the water is absorbed.
3. Remove from heat. Add the cumin and cayenne; stir to blend. Set the pot aside to cool.
4. In a small (1-quart) saucepan, bring ½ cup of water and the bouillon cube to a boil, stirring to dissolve the cube. Add the bulgur. Stir once, cover, and simmer until the broth is absorbed, about 8 minutes. Let stand, covered, to cool.

5. Put the garlic, onion, and olive oil in a large deep-sided skillet. Cook over medium heat, stirring occasionally, until the onions are soft and translucent, about 10 minutes. Add the spinach, cover and cook until wilted, about 3 minutes.
6. Combine the parsley, ½ cup of the feta, eggs, vinegar, salt, and black pepper in a small mixing bowl.
7. In a large mixing bowl, combine the lentils, bulgur, spinach, and feta mixtures. Blend.
8. Transfer to the prepared casserole dish. Arrange the tomato slices on top and garnish with the remaining feta.
9. Bake, uncovered, for 20 minutes.
10. Serve hot or at room temperature with a tossed green salad.

Fried Zucchini Pancakes

Ejjeh

Serves 4

Make this exotic side dish with the cored squash reserved from Fried Stuffed Zucchini (page 157) or start from scratch with fresh zucchini. The recipe calls for a small but potent shot of Arak. Arak is a clear liqueur distilled from grapes with anise. It's imported from Lebanon and sold in liquor stores throughout the United States. Substitute ouzo or sambuca, if you can't find it.

4 small zucchini squash, coarsely grated
¼ cup water
½ teaspoon salt
¼ cup finely chopped onion
¼ cup chopped fresh flat-leaf parsley
1 small clove garlic, pressed
¼ teaspoon ground cumin
¼ teaspoon dried mint
⅛ teaspoon ground black pepper
Pinch of cayenne
1 large egg
1 tablespoon white all-purpose flour
2 teaspoons Arak
Vegetable oil

1. Place the zucchini in a saucepan with the water and salt and cook over moderate heat until tender, about 5 minutes. Drain through a strainer, pressing out excess liquid with a potato masher or fork.
2. Transfer the drained squash to a mixing bowl. Add the onion, parsley, garlic, cumin, mint, black pepper, and cayenne. Mix thoroughly before stirring in the egg, flour, and liqueur.
3. Pour enough vegetable oil in a small skillet so that the oil is about ¼-inch deep. Heat until hot but not smoking. With a large spoon, drop a clump of squash mixture into the hot oil. Fry until golden brown, flipping once,

so that both sides are cooked golden. Drain on paper towels; pat off excess oil, if necessary.

4. These pancakes are tasty served immediately or at room temperature.

☙ Fava Beans in Olive Oil ❧

Foul

Serves 4

Another dish in the collection best known by its Arabic name, foul (pronounced *fool*) is traditionally served surrounded by bowls mounded high with diced fresh tomatoes, finely chopped fresh flat-leaf parsley, and minced scallions. For overnight guests, this can be a special weekend brunch, but we find that the simpler version, without all the extras, makes for a quick, nutritious lunch.

1 can (20 ounces) fava beans, half of the liquid drained off and discarded
Juice of 1 lemon
3 tablespoons extra-virgin olive oil
½ teaspoon salt
½ teaspoon ground cumin
Pinch of cayenne

Garnishes (optional):
2 tomatoes, diced
1 bunch fresh flat-leaf parsley, finely chopped
3 to 4 scallions, finely chopped

1. Place the beans with the remaining half of their liquid, lemon juice, olive oil, salt, cumin, and cayenne in a saucepan. Heat over moderate heat, stirring occasionally, until warmed throughout, about 10 minutes.
2. If desired, chop tomato, parsley, and scallions. Serve each separately in decorative bowls.
3. Spoon individual servings of warmed beans into shallow soup bowls and garnish to taste.

Note: Canned fava beans are sold in Middle Eastern markets and can often be found at your local supermarket in the international foods section.

☙ White Bean Plaki ❧

Serves 4

Plaki is any vegetable dish where you cook the vegetables in olive oil. It can be served hot or cold.

1 cup dried white kidney beans (see Note)
¼ cup olive oil
2 small cloves garlic, finely chopped
2 scallions, finely chopped
¼ cup chopped fresh flat-leaf parsley
1 stalk celery, diced
1 large potato, cut into small cubes
2 carrots, diced
3 tablespoons tomato paste
¼ teaspoon cayenne
1½ teaspoons salt
Juice of ½ lemon
¼ teaspoon ground coriander (optional)

1. Soak the white kidney beans for 4 to 8 hours (overnight) in water. Rinse well and drain.
2. Heat 1 tablespoon of the olive oil in a large deep-sided saucepan. Add garlic and sauté until yellow. Add soaked beans, scallions, parsley, celery, potato, carrots, tomato paste, cayenne, salt, lemon juice, coriander if desired, remaining oil, and 3 cups of water.
3. Bring to a boil. Lower heat and cook, uncovered, until the beans are tender and most of the liquid is absorbed, about 1¼ hours.
4. Delicious served warm or cold.

Note: In most recipes, you can substitute canned beans for dried beans, but not in this recipe, because the cooking time is needed to cook the vegetables as well as the beans.

✑ Cauliflower with Tahini ✑

Serves 4

Quick, easy, delicious—you can't go wrong when you top mild cauliflower florets with the sturdy toasted-nut flavor of tahini. The final dash of cayenne gives this side dish a kick that's irresistible.

1 medium-sized head cauliflower
Salt
¾ cup Tahini Sauce (page 225)
Dash of cayenne

1. Break cauliflower into florets. Wash thoroughly. Bring a pot of salted water to a rapid boil over high heat. Add florets and cook, uncovered, until a fork enters the stems fairly easily, about 10 to 12 minutes.
2. Drain and transfer to a serving bowl. Allow florets to cool slightly before topping with tahini sauce. Toss to mix.
3. Garnish with a dash of cayenne. Serve warm as a side dish.

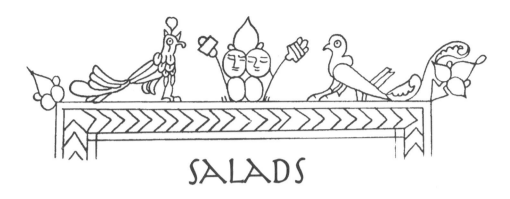

SALADS

⊘ Chickpeas with Spinach ⊘

Nivik

Serves 8

Called nivik in Armenian, this dish can be served warm with bread as a light meal or chilled as a salad. Offer to bring it to your next family gathering or potluck—it's my signature dish. Make it yours, too.

1 large onion, chopped
¼ cup extra-virgin olive oil
¼ cup tomato paste
1¼ teaspoons salt
½ teaspoon ground black pepper
1 teaspoon sugar
1 large bunch fresh flat-leaf parsley, chopped
10 ounces fresh spinach (about 8 cups), washed and roughly chopped, or
1 package (10 ounces) frozen chopped spinach, thawed and pressed dry
2 cans (14½ ounces) chickpeas, drained and rinsed

1. In a large deep-sided skillet, cook the onion in the olive oil over medium heat until tender and translucent, about 10 minutes.
2. Stir in the tomato paste, salt, pepper, sugar, and parsley.
3. Add the spinach and chickpeas. Stir.

4. Add ¼ cup water, cover, and simmer for 15 minutes, stirring occasionally, until spinach is wilted.
5. Remove from heat directly into a serving bowl. Toss before serving.

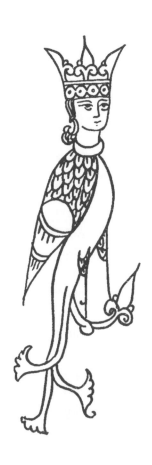

❧ Parsley Salad ❧

Tabouli

Serves 8

Tabouli is a delicate, slightly tart parsley salad whose preparation requires a lot of meticulous chopping in order to get the balance of flavors correct so that it tastes traditional.

½ cup fine-grain bulgur
1½ cups cold water
2 large bunches fresh flat-leaf parsley, very finely chopped (see Note)
1 small sweet onion, finely chopped
1 tablespoon finely chopped fresh mint, or 1 teaspoon dried mint
¼ cup extra-virgin olive oil
Juice of 1 lemon
1 teaspoon salt
½ teaspoon ground black pepper
2 firm ripe tomatoes, diced small

1. Place the bulgur in a bowl and cover with cold water. Stir once to mix, then let soak for 30 minutes. Drain, pressing out excess water. Transfer soaked bulgur to a large serving bowl.
2. Add the parsley, onion, and mint. Toss to combine.
3. In a small bowl, combine the olive oil, lemon juice, salt, and pepper. Pour over the parsley, and toss to cover.
4. Toss in the tomatoes just before serving.
5. Serve at room temperature or chilled with pita slices.

Note: To get light, fluffy parsley, wash and allow it to dry completely before chopping.

❧ Armenian Potato Salad ❧

Serves 8

This simple potato salad has a clean, fresh taste and is best made a day ahead, then served once the flavors have had a chance to blend. It's a perfect alternative for those who want to avoid mayonnaise.

The Salad:
4 large (about 1½ pounds) potatoes, peeled
Salt
3 scallions, diced
1 large bunch fresh flat-leaf parsley, finely chopped

The Dressing:
1 clove garlic, crushed
1 teaspoon salt
¼ teaspoon dried mint
¼ teaspoon ground black pepper
¼ cup lemon juice
¼ cup extra-virgin olive oil
Sprinkle of cayenne (optional)

Special Equipment:
Mortar and pestle

1. Boil the whole, peeled potatoes in enough salted water to cover, until still firm but cooked through, about 25 minutes. Drain and set aside to cool. Cut into bite-sized cubes.
2. Place the potato cubes in a large salad bowl. Add the scallions and parsley.
3. Prepare the dressing by first grinding the garlic and salt into a paste using a mortar and pestle. Transfer the paste to a small mixing bowl and add the mint, black pepper, lemon juice, and olive oil. Whisk briskly.
4. Pour the dressing over the potatoes; toss to coat.
5. Cover with plastic wrap and refrigerate. Garnish with a dash of cayenne, if desired, before serving this salad chilled or at room temperature.

❧ Cracked Wheat–Tomato Salad ❧

Eetch

Serves 8

1 onion, finely chopped
½ green pepper, finely chopped
⅔ cup olive oil
1 can (15 ounces) peeled, diced tomatoes
1 tablespoon tomato paste
1 teaspoon salt
¼ teaspoon ground black pepper
¼ teaspoon cayenne
Juice of 2 lemons
2 cups fine-grain bulgur
1 cup water
Fresh flat-leaf parsley, chopped (optional)
Lettuce or grape leaves

1. Cook onion and green pepper in the olive oil over medium heat until tender, about 10 minutes. Add tomatoes and tomato paste. Simmer, uncovered, for 5 minutes before adding the salt, black pepper, cayenne, and lemon juice. Continue to simmer for 5 more minutes.
2. Remove from heat and transfer to a large mixing bowl. Stir in bulgur and water, mixing well. Let salad sit for 30 minutes before refrigerating.
3. Garnish with parsley, if desired, and serve on a bed of lettuce or cooked grape leaves.

✑ White Bean Salad ↜

Serves 6

White beans make a wonderful canvas for flavorings. The key to obtaining the delicate taste that defines this very Armenian salad is to chop the onion, parsley, and peppers very finely.

The Salad:
2 cans (14½ ounces) white kidney beans, rinsed and drained
¼ cup finely chopped red onion
¼ cup finely chopped fresh flat-leaf parsley
½ red bell pepper, finely chopped
½ green bell pepper, finely chopped

The Dressing:
¼ cup extra-virgin olive oil (see Note)
½ teaspoon salt
¼ teaspoon ground black pepper
¼ teaspoon cayenne
Juice of 2 lemons

1. Combine the beans, onion, parsley, and peppers in a large serving bowl.
2. Whisk the dressing ingredients together until blended. Pour over the beans and toss.
3. This salad is best when served slightly chilled with a generous portion of pita slices.

Note: I always recommend using extra-virgin olive oil for salads and cold dishes because it enhances the flavor of the dish. It's especially important in delicately flavored dishes such as this one.

Cucumber, Tomato, Feta Salad

Serves 8

Use the freshest produce available when making this cooling, elegantly simple salad.

The Salad:
6 firm pickling cucumbers, peeled and diced (about 3 cups)
2 firm, ripe tomatoes, diced (about 2 cups)
¼ pound feta cheese, crumbled (about ¾ cup)
2 tablespoons finely chopped fresh flat-leaf parsley
1 teaspoon snipped fresh chives

The Dressing:
¼ cup extra-virgin olive oil
Juice of 2 lemons

1. Combine the cucumbers, tomatoes, cheese, parsley, and chives in a large salad bowl.
2. Whisk the olive oil with the lemon juice in a small mixing bowl and pour it over the salad. Toss to cover.
3. Serve slightly chilled or at room temperature with grilled meat or poultry and lots of pita.

Cucumber with Yogurt Dressing

Serves 4

This salad is a perfect complement to roasted or grilled lamb.

The Salad:
6 firm pickling cucumbers, peeled and diced (about 3 cups)
1 medium red onion, finely chopped
¼ pound feta cheese, crumbled (about ¾ cup)

The Dressing:
1 cup plain yogurt
1 tablespoon extra-virgin olive oil
Juice of 1 lemon
2 teaspoons chopped fresh mint, or 1 teaspoon dried mint

1. Combine the cucumbers, onion, and cheese in a serving bowl.
2. Place the yogurt in a small bowl and add the olive oil, lemon juice, and mint. Mix well. Pour over the cucumbers and toss to cover.
3. Serve chilled.

✑ Carrots and Toasted Pine Nuts ✑

Serves 6

Carrots are a great year-round root vegetable, but fresh from the garden their sweetness is unbeatable. Look for fairly small, firm, smooth carrots with good color and no cracks or green parts. An extra bonus to eating lots of carrots in the summertime is that they are rich in Vitamin A, a natural sunscreen vitamin.

The Salad:
1 pound (6 - 7) carrots, shredded (about 3 cups)
1 cup Toasted Pine Nuts (page 43)

The Dressing:
¼ cup extra-virgin olive oil
Juice of 1 lemon
½ teaspoon salt
2 teaspoons chopped fresh mint, or ½ teaspoon dried mint
1 teaspoon snipped fresh dill, or ¼ teaspoon dried dill

1. Combine the carrot and pine nuts in a serving bowl.
2. In a small mixing bowl, whisk the dressing ingredients together. Pour over the carrots and toss to cover.
3. Serve at room temperature or slightly chilled.

✑ Beet and Walnut Salad ✒

Serves 8

The Salad:
3 medium beets, stems removed and discarded
1 cup finely chopped walnuts

The Dressing:
1 very small clove garlic
½ teaspoon salt
3 tablespoons red wine vinegar

Special Equipment:
Mortar and pestle

1. In a large saucepan with enough water to cover, boil whole beets for 30 minutes or until firm, but not soft. Drain and cool before peeling.
2. Shred the peeled beets with a grater into a mixing bowl. Stir in walnuts.
3. Mash garlic and salt into a paste in a mortar and pestle. Go light on the garlic. If you don't, it will quickly overpower the other flavors in the dish.
4. Transfer the garlic paste to a small mixing bowl. Add the vinegar and mix well before adding to the beets. Toss to coat.
5. This salad is pretty when offered as individual servings over a bed of lettuce on small salad plates.

᪥ Swiss Chard with Tahini ᪥

Serves 4

Swiss chard is one of the most popular leafy greens of the Mediterranean. Honoring that popularity with a special place in their cuisine, Armenians traditionally make and serve this salad on Easter Eve as the final dish of Lent.

The Salad:
1 bunch fresh Swiss chard
1 large bunch fresh flat-leaf parsley, chopped

The Dressing:
¾ cup Tahini Sauce (page 225)

1. Wash the Swiss chard; cut off and discard stems. Finely chop the leaves.
2. Bring 1 cup of water to a boil in a large deep-sided skillet, add the leaves, cover, and simmer gently for 2 minutes. Remove from heat and keep covered for another 2 minutes. Drain, pressing out excess liquid.
3. Transfer the chard to a salad bowl. Cool to room temperature before adding the parsley. Toss, cover with plastic wrap, and refrigerate.
4. Serve chilled, drizzled with tahini sauce.

✑ Stuffed Tomatoes ✑

Serves 8

8 large tomatoes
1¼ teaspoons salt
2 tablespoons red lentils, picked clean of debris and rinsed
1 onion, finely chopped
2 tablespoons olive oil
½ cup coarse-grain bulgur
1 pound fresh Swiss chard or spinach (about 13 cups), stems discarded
and leaves finely chopped
¼ teaspoon ground black pepper
¼ cup Toasted Pine Nuts (page 43)
½ cup dried currants
⅓ cup chopped fresh flat-leaf parsley
1 teaspoon snipped fresh dill
Juice of 2 lemons

1. Cut off the top third of each tomato and scoop out insides, leaving shells intact for stuffing. Transfer the pulp to a sieve set over a bowl to drain excess liquid. (Chop the drained tomato pulp and use in Vegetable Medley [page 66]. Chop the tomato tops and use for Cucumber, Tomato, Feta Salad [page 89].)
2. Sprinkle the insides of the tomato shells with ½ teaspoon salt and drain upside-down on a rack set in a pan while you prepare the filling. (You can prepare the tomato shells the day before. Just cover the draining shells tightly with plastic wrap and refrigerate.)
3. Simmer the lentils in ½ cup water in a small saucepan until just tender, about 20 minutes. Drain, rinse under cold water, and drain again before setting aside.
4. Cook the onion in the oil over moderate heat in a large deep-sided skillet, stirring occasionally, until tender, about 10 minutes. Add the bulgur, chard or spinach, remaining ¾ teaspoon salt, and pepper. Cook, stirring, until greens wilt, about 2 minutes. Add 1 cup of water, then remove from heat and let stand, covered, until the bulgur softens, about 30 minutes.

5. Transfer to a large mixing bowl and stir in the pine nuts, currants, parsley, dill, lemon juice, and lentils.
6. Spoon filling into the tomato shells.
7. Serve at room temperature with Vegetable Medley (page 66) and your choice of a meat or poultry dish. Roast Pork Stuffed with Shallots and Apricots (page 174) is an excellent choice.

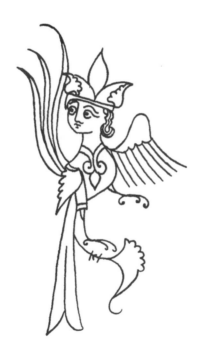

❧ Potato and Chickpea Salad ❧

Serves 8

Thankfully, when it's summertime and you are living through a heat wave, Armenian cooking adapts well to record-breaking temperatures. This salad complements any grilled meat and its zesty flavor tastes even better as the flavors blend. So make it in the cool of the evening and relish it chilled in the heat of the day.

The Salad:
6 large (about 2 pounds) potatoes, peeled
Salt
2 cans (14½ ounces) chickpeas, drained and rinsed
3 scallions, finely chopped
1 bunch fresh flat-leaf parsley, finely chopped

The Dressing:
½ cup extra-virgin olive oil
¼ cup balsamic vinegar
1 teaspoon dry mustard
1 teaspoon salt
½ teaspoon ground black pepper

1. Boil the peeled potatoes whole in a large pot of salted water with the cover cracked until the potatoes are firm but cooked through, about 25 minutes. Remove from heat and drain. Set aside to cool.
2. Cut the potatoes into bite-sized cubes, transfer to a large serving bowl, and toss in the chickpeas, scallions, and parsley.
3. Combine the dressing ingredients in a small mixing bowl. Whisk briskly. Slowly pour about ¾ of the dressing over the salad, stirring to coat. Add more if necessary, but be careful not to float the salad in dressing. (Excess dressing may be saved and used within the next few days to dress a tossed green salad.)
4. Cover and chill. Allow the flavors to blend for at least 2 hours before serving.

✑ Four-Bean Salad ✑

Often called "the food of the poor" or "peasant food," bean dishes are full of fiber, wholesome, and filling as well as inexpensive. This salad is a crowd pleaser.

The Salad:
1 can (14½ ounces) chickpeas, drained and rinsed
1 can (14½ ounces) red kidney beans, drained and rinsed
1 can (14½ ounces) white kidney beans, drained and rinsed
1 can (15 ounces) black beans, drained and rinsed
1 small red onion, thinly sliced
1 large bunch fresh flat-leaf parsley, chopped

The Dressing:
½ cup extra-virgin olive oil
¼ cup balsamic vinegar
Juice of 1 lemon
½ teaspoon ground cumin
½ teaspoon salt
¼ teaspoon cayenne

1. Combine the beans, onion, and parsley in a large serving bowl.
2. In a small mixing bowl, whisk the dressing ingredients until blended; then pour over the beans. Toss to coat.
3. Serve chilled or at room temperature. Offer as one of a medley of salads for a complete meal.

❧ Bulgur Salad with Chickpeas and Greens ❧

Serves 8

This is a robust, flavorful, do-ahead salad dressed with spicy seasonings. The spinach, parsley, and scallions paint a medley of greens when mixed with the warm brown of the nutty-flavored cracked wheat. Serve with a wholesome soup for a meal that will warm you up and cool you down—much like the New England weather in March.

The Salad:
1 cup medium-grain bulgur
2 cups water, boiling
10 ounces fresh spinach (about 8 cups), washed
2 scallions, diced
1 small bunch fresh flat-leaf parsley, chopped
1 can (14½ ounces) chickpeas, drained and rinsed

The Dressing:
1 small clove garlic, pressed
⅓ cup extra-virgin olive oil
Juice of 1 lemon
2 tablespoons red wine vinegar
½ teaspoon ground cumin
¼ teaspoon cayenne
½ teaspoon salt

1. Place the bulgur in a large serving bowl. Stir in the boiling water and let stand for at least 30 minutes or until the water is fully absorbed. This method helps produce bulgur that is light and fluffy.
2. Bring ¼ cup water to a boil in a large deep-sided skillet. Add the spinach and simmer, covered, for 2 minutes or until spinach wilts. Drain and press out excess moisture before transferring to a work surface. Chop fine, stir in the bulgur, and transfer to a large mixing bowl. Add the scallions, parsley, and chickpeas, tossing to mix.

3. Combine all of the dressing ingredients in a small bowl and mix well. Drizzle over the salad. Toss thoroughly. Cover and chill.
4. For maximum visual effect, serve individual portions on a small bed of Romaine lettuce.

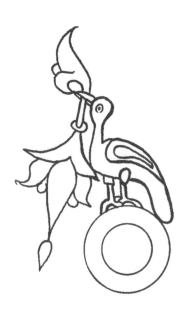

❧ Zahtar-Spiced Pasta Salad ❧

Serves 4

Pasta is not a staple in the Middle East like it is in the West. My husband created this recipe when he first came to the United States. As a single guy working long hours, he needed an easy salad which tasted like home that he could prepare ahead and have in the refrigerator. Zahtar is the herb that makes this pasta salad so different. It is an olive-green, tangy blend containing a thyme-like herb (called zahtar in the Middle East), sumac bark, and sesame seeds. It's imported from Lebanon and Syria.

My husband recommends eating this salad straight—pasta with dressing. I'm the one who tends to toss in optional items. Any way you chose to make it, it is unique and tasty, and perfect for outdoor eating events like barbecues and picnics.

The Salad:
1 pound twisted rainbow pasta (substitute eggless pasta if fasting)

The Dressing:
2 - 3 tablespoons extra-virgin olive oil
1 tablespoon balsamic vinegar
Juice of 1 lemon
2 tablespoons zahtar
1½ teaspoons dried mint
¼ teaspoon ground cumin
¼ teaspoon oregano
¼ teaspoon thyme
½ teaspoon salt

Additions (Optional):
Feta cheese, crumbled
Black olives, pitted and chopped
Tomatoes, diced
Celery, diced
Fresh flat-leaf parsley, chopped

1. Cook the pasta according to the instructions on the package. Drain, rinse well, and place in a large salad bowl.
2. In a small mixing bowl, combine the dressing ingredients, whisking until well blended. Pour the dressing over the pasta and toss until covered.
3. Serve as is or get creative and add any one or more of the additional ingredients listed, or anything else you might have in the refrigerator!

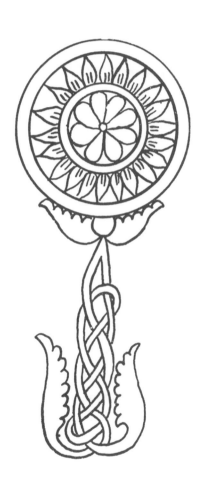

❧ Purslane and Fresh Tomatoes ❧

Serves 4

Purslane, called per-per in Armenian, can sometimes be found at farmers' markets and often in your own yard or garden! It is a trailing weed with fleshy reddish stems and small succulent leaves and is best eaten after blanching, which gives it a savory lemon flavor.

This recipe was handed down to me from my cousin, who learned to make it from our grandmother, who would forage for per-per in her huge garden. My cousin was the first houseguest at our home in Rhode Island. As I was giving him the penny-tour of the yard, he stopped short, pointed to a sprawling patch of weeds, and shouted, "That's per-per! Grandma used to make a salad out of that." Without hesitation, he picked a substantial bunch and contributed this salad to our barbecue that evening.

This salad offers the delicate and intense flavors of a traditional herb salad and is a delicious complement to any summer meal.

The Salad:
2 cups purslane, washed (see Note)
1 large bunch fresh flat-leaf parsley, finely chopped
1 medium-sized firm, ripe tomato, diced
1 small red onion, sliced thin

The Dressing:
¼ cup extra-virgin olive oil
Juice of 1 lemon
1 small clove garlic, pressed
½ teaspoon salt
¼ teaspoon sumac

1. Bring 3 cups water to a boil in a medium-sized saucepan. Plunge the purslane into the boiling water and cook until the plant wilts and the red from the stems bleeds into the liquid, about 7 minutes. Remove from heat and immediately rinse under cold running water. Drain.
2. Combine the purslane, parsley, tomato, and onion in a serving bowl.

3. Whisk the olive oil, lemon juice, garlic, salt, and sumac together in a small bowl. Pour over the salad and toss.

Note: Substitute fresh finely chopped baby spinach and finely shredded Romaine lettuce for purslane with good effect. The secret is to cut each leaf as thinly as possible, then mix the greens together ahead of time so they wilt some and the flavors mix. Toss in dressing just before serving to keep the greens from expressing too much moisture. This is especially important the more salt the dressing contains.

☜ Spinach Salad with Fava Beans ☞

Serves 4

Fava beans are an excellent source of fiber. When paired with spinach, they makes a salad that is as good for you as it is appetizing.

The Salad:
1 pound fresh spinach (about 13 cups), washed and chopped
1 can (20 ounces) fava beans, drained and rinsed
¼ cup thinly sliced red onion
¼ cup finely chopped fresh flat-leaf parsley

The Dressing:
2 tablespoons extra-virgin olive oil
Juice of 1 lemon
¼ teaspoon salt
¼ teaspoon ground black pepper

1. Place the spinach, fava beans, onion, and parsley in a large serving bowl.
2. Whisk the olive oil, lemon juice, salt, and black pepper together in a small mixing bowl.
3. Pour the dressing over the greens and toss to cover.

Note: Today, canned fava beans can often be found in your local supermarket.

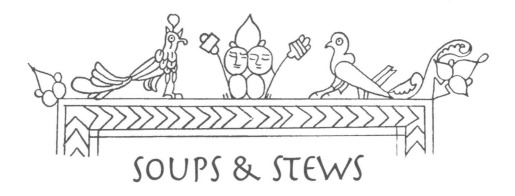

SOUPS & STEWS

Chilled Yogurt Soup with Cucumbers

Jajek

Serves 2

Beat the heat on a hot summer day with this super-simple, no-cook, thirst-quenching, yogurt-based soup. Second only to pilaf, jajek is an Armenian staple.

1 large firm cucumber, peeled
1 cup plain yogurt
½ teaspoon salt
1 tablespoon finely chopped fresh mint
1 cup ice cold water (see Note)

1. Cut the cucumber in half lengthwise. Remove and discard seeds. Cut each half lengthwise again, then dice each section into small pieces, the tinier the tastier.
2. Combine the chopped cucumber, yogurt, salt, mint, and water in a ceramic or glass bowl. Mix well. Cover and chill.
3. Feast on an individual serving of this delicious soup.

Note: For a special treat, omit the water, and spoon over pilaf, grilled lamb, or rounds of grilled eggplant as a condiment.

✑ Lentil and Swiss Chard Soup ✑

Serves 4

Midwinter is the season for hearty soups and home-baked breads. A thick slice of Cracked Wheat Bread (page 199) with a bowl of this soup is truly satisfying.

1½ cups brown lentils, picked clean of debris and rinsed
10 leaves Swiss chard, washed, stems removed and discarded
¼ cup olive oil
1 large onion, finely chopped
1 large clove garlic, finely chopped
¼ cup chopped fresh flat-leaf parsley
1 teaspoon salt
½ teaspoon ground black pepper
Juice of 2 lemons

1. Place the lentils in a large pot with 6 cups cold water. Bring to a boil, skimming off any foam that emerges, then cover and simmer gently for 1 hour or until lentils are soft but not mushy.
2. Slit the Swiss chard leaves down the middle and chop coarsely. The taste is the same whether you use red or green chard. I love colorful food, so I use a combination of both.
3. Heat the olive oil in a large deep-sided skillet; add the onion and garlic and sauté gently until the onion is tender and transparent, about 10 minutes. Add the shredded chard leaves. Stirring frequently, cook until the leaves wilt, about 5 minutes.
4. Pour the skillet mixture into the lentils. Add the parsley, salt, pepper, and lemon juice. Cover and simmer gently for 15 minutes.
5. Serve with extra lemon wedges, if desired, and hearty slices of bread and cheese to complete the meal.

☙ Red Lentil Soup ❧

Vospov Abour

Serves 8

This soup is an old-time favorite made in some version by just about every nationality of cooks from the Middle East. Red lentils are light and cook quickly, so it is a particularly good soup to be able to pull out of your chef's hat year-round.

1 garlic clove, minced
1 small onion, finely chopped
3 tablespoons olive oil
2 cups red lentils, picked clean of debris and rinsed
5 cups chicken or vegetable broth
½ teaspoon ground cardamom
½ teaspoon salt

1. In a skillet, sauté the garlic and onion in the olive oil over moderate heat until the onions are tender, about 10 minutes.
2. Place the lentils in a large pot. Add the onion mixture, the broth, cardamon, and salt. Bring the soup to a boil; reduce heat, cover, and simmer until the lentils become soft and mushy, about 45 minutes. When done, the soup will be golden yellow and the lentils will have broken up so that individual lentils are rare.
3. Traditionally served warm topped with Toasted Pita Chips (page 191).

❦ Brown Lentil Soup ❧

Serves 4

2 cups brown lentils, picked clean of debris and rinsed
1 large onion, finely chopped
1 whole bay leaf (preferably Turkish)
¾ teaspoon salt

The Topping:
2 - 4 (8-inch) pita rounds
¼ cup olive oil

1. Soak the lentils in cold water for at least 1 hour. Drain and rinse well under cold running water.
2. Place the soaked lentils, onion, bay leaf, and 4 cups water in a medium-sized saucepan. Cover and bring to a boil over high heat, then lower the heat and simmer for about 20 minutes or until the lentils are tender. Stir in the salt. Remove and discard the bay leaf.
3. As the soup simmers, slice or tear the pita rounds into single-layer, bite-sized pieces. Heat the oil in a medium-sized skillet until hot but not smoking. Fry the pita pieces in the olive oil until brown and crispy. Remove with a slotted spoon and drain on paper towels.
4. Top individual soup servings with a small handful of the fried bread.

❧ Yellow Split-Pea Soup ❧

Serves 6

1 pound yellow split-peas
1 vegetable bouillon cube
½ onion, finely chopped
2 tablespoons olive oil
½ teaspoon salt
¼ teaspoon ground cumin
¼ teaspoon ground black pepper
Pinch of cayenne

1. Rinse the peas under cold running water, then place them in a large saucepan. Add 7½ cups of water and the bouillon cube. Bring to a boil. Stir frequently until the cube dissolves and skim off any white foam that collects on top with a spoon, then lower heat and simmer, partially covered, for 35 minutes.
2. As the peas simmer, sauté the onion in the olive oil in a skillet over moderate heat until the onion is tender, about 10 minutes.
3. Add the cooked onion, salt, cumin, and peppers, stirring well to mix. Continue to simmer another 10 minutes or until the peas lose their shape and disintegrate.
4. Serve hot with a generous portion of Toasted Pita Chips (page 191).

Red Pepper Soup

Serves 4

Armenians love peppers. My grandmother grew all kinds in the huge garden she kept behind her house.

One weekend when I was visiting, my cousin was sick. I spent most of the day playing cards with him, but by suppertime we were getting restless and bored. So my grandmother asked us to help her remove the stems and seeds from a basket filled with beautiful, long, thin red peppers from the garden. Not long later, the skin around our eyes, nostrils, and mouths began burning. We started to scream and cry. We thought we were on fire! Grandma had asked us to core hot peppers! We spent the next hour with our heads stuck under running water to dilute the flaming pepper juice that had soaked into our skin.

I share this story with you because after roasting, the serranos may seem small, but they are the little firecrackers that add just the right amount of hot to the sweet base of this soup to send your senses soaring. Serve as an aperitif or alongside a stuffed pastry borek as a complete meal that meets all the known and conceivable requirements of "gourmet."

4 medium-sized sweet red peppers, cut in half lengthwise
2 small green serrano peppers
2 large cloves garlic
1 tablespoon olive oil
1 can (14½ ounces) chicken broth (see Note)
½ cup light whipping cream
Fresh tarragon snips

Special Equipment:
Food processor

1. Preheat the oven to 425 degrees.
2. Remove the stems, membranes, and seeds from the peppers. Place the peppers, cut side down, and the garlic on a foil-lined baking sheet. Brush the peppers and garlic with olive oil. Bake for 20 to 25 minutes or until

the pepper skins are bubbly. Remove from the oven and place peppers in a bag until just cool. Remove skins from peppers and garlic.

3. Place the roasted red and serrano peppers and the garlic in a saucepan and add the broth. Bring to a boil, reduce heat and simmer, uncovered, for about 7 minutes or until the liquid is reduced by one-third. Set aside to cool slightly.

4. Place the cooked pepper mixture in the bowl of a food processor and blend until smooth. Transfer the mixture back into the same saucepan. Stir in the cream. Cook and stir until the soup is heated through.

6. Ladle into individual serving bowls. Top with tarragon snips and serve immediately.

Note: Vegetarians may substitute vegetable broth without compromising taste.

Homemade Chicken Broth

Makes 8 cups

In frugal kitchens, it is considered wasteful to discard anything. Honoring the ancient culinary roots of my ancestors, I save all chicken bones, wings, backs, gizzards, and scraps in the freezer until I have enough to make a homemade stock. Whenever I have the time, I make a big pot of broth and freeze containers that hold 1½ cups (12 ounces), so that I have it on hand, pre-measured to make pilaf.

8 cups raw and/or cooked chicken bones and scraps
2 teaspoons salt

1. Put the bones and scraps into a large (3-quart) pot. Add enough water to cover the chicken by 1 inch, about 10 cups. Add salt and bring to a simmer. A grayish scum will come to the surface. Skim it occasionally until it stops forming.
2. Cover the pot. Simmer 1½ hours.
3. Allow to cool, then strain the broth. Now you may discard the chicken parts. Cover and refrigerate. The next day, remove the fat congealed on the surface if you want a low fat broth or distribute it evenly among your containers for a tastier bouillon with more body. Keep refrigerated or freeze.

◦⟨ Bulgur Stew with Chickpeas ⟩◦

Serves 8

This hearty vegetarian stew will take the chill out of the bitterest winter day.

3 tablespoons olive oil
1¼ cup coarse-grain bulgur
1 medium onion, finely chopped
1 - 2 cloves garlic, finely chopped
3 celery stalks, diced
2 cans (14½ ounces) tomatoes, peeled and diced
1½ cups cold water
2 cans (14 ounces) chickpeas, drained and rinsed
1 teaspoon sugar
½ teaspoon ground cumin
⅛ teaspoon cayenne
½ teaspoon ground black pepper
1 teaspoon salt

1. Heat the oil in a large saucepan. Add the bulgur, onion, and garlic and sauté for 5 minutes over medium-high heat, stirring frequently. Add the celery and cook for a few more minutes.
2. Add the tomatoes, water, chickpeas, sugar, cumin, peppers, and salt. Stir well. Cover and simmer, stirring occasionally, until most of the liquid has been absorbed, about 20 to 25 minutes. The bulgur will be plump and tender when the stew is done.
3. Serve warm with a delicious flatbread and a slice of cheese.

Tomato and Bulgur Soup

Serves 4

My husband calls this soup "healing soup" because his father requested it whenever he was feeling a bit under the weather. This home remedy may not be a medically proven cure, but its rich, hearty flavor and wholesome warmth will improve your spirits.

6 cups chicken broth
½ onion, very finely chopped
2 tablespoons olive oil
1 can (6 ounces) tomato paste (about ¾ cup)
1 cup fine-grain bulgur
1 teaspoon salt
¾ teaspoon ground black pepper
1 lemon

1. Bring broth to a boil over moderate-high heat in a large pot.
2. Meanwhile, sauté the onion in the olive oil in a small saucepan over moderate heat until tender and slightly golden brown, about 10 minutes.
3. Add the tomato paste to the boiling broth. Stir until the paste is distributed evenly before adding the bulgur, salt, and pepper. Stir to combine, then add the cooked onion. Cover, lower heat, and simmer for 10 minutes.
4. Serve individually in bowls with a squeeze of fresh lemon.

Cold Yogurt Barley Soup

Serves 4

The creation of this classic yogurt soup is credited to the regions of Eastern Anatolia around Erzurum and Van, but all Armenian families have adopted one version or another of the recipe. This is my grandmother's recipe. Version 1 is cold; Version 2 is hot. Either way, it's nutritious and yummy.

1 cup pearl barley
Salt
2 tablespoons finely chopped onion
1 small clove garlic, pressed
2 large cucumbers, peeled, seeded, and finely chopped
1 tablespoon finely chopped fresh mint, or 1 - 1½ teaspoons dried mint
4 cups (2 pounds) plain yogurt
2 cups cold water
½ teaspoon salt
Dash of cayenne
Ice cubes (optional)

1. In a large saucepan, cover the barley with approximately 3 cups water and a dash of salt. Bring to a boil. Reduce heat, and simmer, until barley is soft, about 40 minutes. Drain, rinse well with cold water, drain again, and set aside until cool.
2. Combine the barley, onion, garlic, cucumbers, and mint in a large bowl. Stir in the yogurt, then slowly add the cold water. Continue stirring to create a thin, creamy mix before adding the salt and cayenne.
3. Chill thoroughly. Serve in bowls with a few ice cubes added, if desired.

Hot Yogurt Barley Soup

Serves 4

1 cup pearl barley
6 cups chicken or vegetable broth
1 large onion, finely chopped
1 tablespoon butter
½ cup chopped fresh flat-leaf parsley
1 tablespoon chopped fresh mint, or 1 - 1½ teaspoons dried mint
¾ teaspoon salt
½ teaspoon ground black pepper
4 cups (2 pounds) plain yogurt
1 large egg
Juice of 1 lemon

1. Place the barley in a large bowl with enough cold water to cover, and soak the kernels for 4 to 8 hours (overnight). Drain, rinse well with cold water, and drain again.
2. Place the soaked barley in a large pot with the broth.
3. In a separate skillet, sauté the onions in the butter over moderate heat, until golden, about 10 minutes. Then stir them into the broth.
4. Add the parsley, mint, salt, and pepper. Bring the soup to a boil, lower heat, and simmer, covered, for 1½ hours.
5. Approximately 10 minutes before the end of the cooking time given in step 4, beat the yogurt, egg, and lemon juice in a small mixing bowl until smooth. Then add the yogurt to the soup, stirring continuously, until the broth is creamy.
6. Best served at once, very hot.

Ground Lamb and Zucchini Soup

Serves 6

This soup is a culinary inspiration shared by my husband's aunt, who lives in Cairo, Egypt. Auntie Arak contributed it to a family cookbook we published in the mid-1990s. Since then it has become a staple in our house, and many American guests at our table have raved that this soup "is to die for." While I'm not sure this popular American cliché describing great taste would be fully understood in Egypt, I do know that Auntie Arak's soup qualifies as one of the most delicious soups on the planet.

3 medium zucchini, diced
1 onion, finely chopped
1 teaspoon salt
½ teaspoon ground black pepper
5 tablespoons white all-purpose flour
1 tablespoon olive oil
6 - 7 cups chicken broth
½ pound very lean (95% lean) ground lamb (kheyma meat)
1 - 2 lemons, cut in wedges

1. Combine the zucchini and onion in a large bowl, season with salt and pepper, and sprinkle 3 tablespoons of flour evenly over the top. Toss until all pieces are covered.
2. Combine the olive oil and the remaining 2 tablespoons flour in a large pot. Stir into a paste.
3. In a second large pot, heat the chicken broth over moderate heat, then transfer 2 cups of heated broth to the pot with the paste, stirring until the paste dissolves. Add the remaining broth and bring to a boil.
4. Add the zucchini and onion to the boiling broth. Reduce heat and simmer, covered, for about 15 minutes. Then add the meat, breaking it up as you add it. Stir well, cover, and continue to simmer for another 15 minutes.
5. Serve in individual soup bowls with a squeeze of fresh lemon.

Barley Mash with Chicken

Herisa

Serves a small army

The Lenten fast is broken with soup called herisa. To this day, in church halls across America, parishioners join to eat large bowls of this barley mash in celebration of Easter. I recommend that, if you want to try this soup, join your local church feast, because making it at home, even without the elbow grease, is somewhat of an ordeal, and honestly, it's an acquired taste.

The Soup:
3 cups pearl barley
1 gallon (4 quarts) cold water
2 teaspoons salt
1 teaspoon ground black pepper
1 small (2- to 4-pound) roaster chicken, innards removed
3 hours of elbow grease (optional)

The Toppings:
¼ pound (1 stick) butter, melted
Ground cumin

1. Soak the barley for 4 to 8 hours (overnight) in cold water. Drain and rinse.
2. In a very large pot, season water with salt and black pepper and bring to a boil. Gently lower the chicken (whole) into the boiling water, lower heat, and simmer, covered, for 1½ hours or until the chicken is very well done. Remove the bird to a work surface to cool, leaving the broth in the pot.
3. Once cooled, remove the chicken meat from the bones, discarding the bones and skin. Shred the meat as finely as possible. Place the shredded chicken back into the broth and add the soaked barley.
4. Simmer over low heat, uncovered, stirring occasionally, for about 30 minutes or until the barley soaks up all the broth.

5. At this point, the traditional method of preparing this soup calls for the cook to beat the mixture with a wooden spoon for at least 3 hours, until it becomes a uniform paste. (Forget that!) Instead beat the soup with an electric mixer until it resembles oatmeal mush, about 20 minutes.

6. Serve in individual serving bowls drizzled with a spoonful of melted butter and a sprinkle of cumin on top.

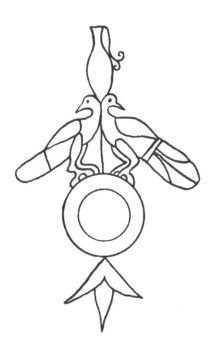

❧ Vegetable Herisa ❧

Serves 4

I have never been too successful making traditional herisa—a thick soup of barley and meat, usually chicken or lamb. No matter what recipe I followed, it came out tasting like paste and ended up lumping in my stomach. I gave up on herisa until presented with the challenge of coming up with a new Lenten dish for the weekly newspaper column I wrote that became the basis for this book. When I started to play with a vegetarian version, I discovered that veggies blend and balance beautifully with barley. Here's an original herisa recipe I can recommend.

The Soup:
1½ cups pearl barley
1 teaspoon dried mint
½ teaspoon ground cumin
2 teaspoons salt
¼ teaspoon ground black pepper
3 - 4 carrots, shredded (about 1½ cups)
1 small zucchini, diced (about 1½ cups)
3 stalks celery, diced (about 1½ cups)

The Toppings:
4 tablespoons (½ stick) butter, melted (omit if fasting)
Sprinkle of cayenne

1. Soak the barley for 4 to 8 hours (overnight) in enough water to cover. Rinse well and drain.
2. Combine the barley, mint, cumin, salt, and pepper with 3 cups water in a large pot. Bring it to a boil over high heat.
3. Add the carrots, zucchini, and celery. Lower the heat and simmer, uncovered, until the barley soaks up all the water, about 20 minutes. The stew will thicken like oatmeal.
4. Serve individual portions in soup bowls, garnished with a generous spoonful of melted butter and a dash of cayenne.

Yogurt Soup with Harpout Kuftehs

Serves 6

My Harpout Kufteh recipe works especially well when making this soup because I use fresh uncooked parsley in the filling, so little green parsley flakes float out of the center of the kuftehs as you eat the soup—a fresh, colorful, and tasty surprise.

8 cups chicken broth
12 Harpout Kuftehs, prepared as described on page 152
4 cups (2 pounds) plain yogurt
1 large egg
Juice of 1 lemon
Dash of cayenne or sumac (optional)

1. Place the chicken broth in a large pot and bring to a simmer. Add the kuftehs.
2. Immediately beat the yogurt, egg, and lemon juice in a bowl until smooth. Then add 1 ladle of chicken broth at a time to the yogurt, stirring continuously. After transferring about 5 ladles of broth, pour the warmed yogurt into the soup. Continue stirring and bring to a boil over moderate heat.
3. Serve piping hot, garnished with a dash of cayenne or sumac, if desired.

Lamb and Rhubarb Stew

Serves 4

Make this savory stew with both spring and fall rhubarb harvests.

1 pound lamb stew meat
1 medium-sized onion, chopped
2 tablespoons butter
3 cups rhubarb, diced
2 tablespoons sugar
1 bunch fresh flat-leaf parsley, chopped
3 cups water
½ teaspoon ground cinnamon
½ teaspoon ground nutmeg
1 teaspoon salt
½ teaspoon ground black pepper

1. Brown the meat in a deep-sided skillet. Add 2 to 3 cups water. The water level should be high enough to cover the meat chunks slightly more than halfway. Cover and simmer for 1 hour. Cool. Remove the cooked meat from the bone and place the meat chunks in a large saucepan.
2. Add the butter, rhubarb, sugar, parsley, water, and spices; stir to mix. Bring to a boil, reduce heat, cover, and simmer for 45 minutes.
3. Serve this light stew over pilaf or a bed of mashed potatoes.

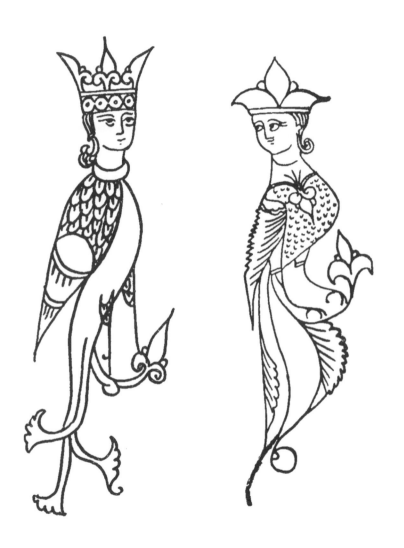

STUFFED PASTRIES (BOREKS)

Folding Phyllo Triangles

Borek is the Turkish word for pie. Most often, dough is stuffed with the chef's favorite center—sometimes a blend of cheeses, spinach, or spiced meats—and folded into triangles. The triangles are served as a prelude to a meal, as a side dish, and sometimes even for dessert with coffee. Folding triangles takes more time than cutting a pan-layered borek into squares, so I don't fold triangle-shaped boreks often. But for the traditionalists in the group, here's how.

1. Remove the phyllo from its packaging (see Glossary, page 284). Cover the stack of dough with 2 overlapping sheets of plastic wrap topped with a clean, dampened kitchen towel. This will keep the dough from drying out until you are ready to use it.
2. Take 1 sheet from the stack and arrange it on a work surface with a long side nearest you and brush it with melted butter. Place another sheet on top and brush with more butter. Cut the buttered layers crosswise (vertical; from top to bottom) into 6 (roughly 12 x 2¾-inch) strips.
3. Put a heaping teaspoon of filling near the corner of a strip, at the end nearest you or farthest from you. Fold a corner of phyllo over the stuffing to enclose the filling and form a triangle. Continue folding the strip (like

a flag), maintaining the triangle shape. When folded, brush the seam with melted butter to secure it, then place the triangle, seam side down, on a large baking sheet and brush the top with butter. Repeat until all the phyllo sheets have been folded into triangles.

4. Preheat the oven to 350 degrees. Bake the triangles until golden brown, about 20 to 25 minutes.

5. Transfer the triangles to a wire rack to cool slightly before serving.

Note: To freeze, place a single layer of stuffed triangles in the bottom of a freezer-proof container. Place the container in the freezer just long enough for the butter to harden, then lay more triangles on top and freeze again. Chilling one layer at a time prevents the boreks from sticking together. Another way is to separate each layer with a sheet of waxed paper. When guests arrive, remove as many frozen triangles as you need and bake them on cookie sheets in a preheated 350 degree oven for 20 minutes or until golden, turning once during baking to ensure even browning on both sides.

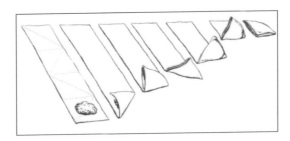

Cheese Borek

Makes 24

The best way to cut down on holiday kitchen stress is to prepare a few dishes ahead of time and freeze them.

Martha Saraydarian, an excellent home cook, who entertains extended family often, shared this recipe with me along with freezing tips, so you, too, will be prepared when hungry company arrives. Thanks, Martha!

The Filling:
1 pound Muenster cheese, shredded
1 cup small-curd cottage cheese (for best results, use
2% - 4% fat cheese)
1 teaspoon baking powder
1 bunch fresh flat-leaf parsley, finely chopped
2 large eggs, beaten

The Shell:
1 package phyllo dough (see Glossary, page 284)
⅜ pound (1½ sticks) butter, melted

1. Combine the two cheeses, baking powder, parsley, and eggs in a large mixing bowl.
2. Preheat the oven to 350 degrees.
3. Remove the phyllo dough from its packaging. Cover immediately with 2 overlapping sheets of plastic wrap and a clean, slightly moistened kitchen towel to prevent the dough from drying before use.
4. Brush the bottom of the baking tray with butter. Lay 1 phyllo sheet in the buttered tray. Working quickly, brush it with butter and lay a second layer of dough; repeat until you have 10 sheets in the tray.
5. Spread the cheese mixture evenly over the phyllo and layer 10 more sheets of dough, buttering between each sheet as before. Brush the top of the finished pie with butter and, with a sharp knife, cut into squares, about 3 x 3-inches in size.

6. Bake in the middle of the oven for about 25 minutes, or until the top is golden brown.
7. Martha serves these savory treats with coffee as dessert, but I serve them at parties as an appetizer or with a tossed green salad for a light meal.

Note: To freeze, cover the assembled, uncooked borek in the baking tray with plastic wrap then foil and place in the freezer. Defrost tray completely before baking.

Four-Cheese Pasta Borek

Serves 10

This is another recipe that serves ten people or more, gets rave reviews from all ages, and freezes well.

Feel free to play with the combination of cheeses. In my kitchen we use the sweet white cheese from Syria if we are on the East Coast and the common, easy-to-find white cheese from Mexico if we are on the West Coast. A mild Swiss or Gruyere works, too. Or change the mix completely and use whatever you have in the refrigerator.

The Filling:
¾ package (1 pound) wide egg (lasagna) noodles
1 cup shredded sharp white cheddar cheese
1 cup shredded mozzarella cheese
1 cup shredded white sweet cheese
½ cup crumbled feta cheese
1 large bunch fresh flat-leaf parsley, finely chopped
½ teaspoon ground black pepper
1 small onion, finely chopped
¼ pound (1 stick) unsalted butter, melted

The Shell:
1 package (2 sheets) frozen puff pastry sheet dough (see Note)
White all-purpose flour for rolling
1 large egg, beaten

1. Preheat the oven to 350 degrees.
2. Cook the noodles according to the package instructions. Drain and set them aside.
3. Combine the cheeses, parsley, milk, pepper, onion, and butter in a large bowl. Mix well.
4. Using a rolling pin, roll 1 of the pastry sheets out on a floured work surface to fit the size of the tray. Lay the pastry sheet on the bottom of the prepared tray.

5. Cover the dough with 1 layer of cooked noodles. Spread the cheese mixture evenly over the noodles. Cover the cheese with another layer of noodles. Roll out the remaining pastry sheet and place it on top.

6. Tuck the top dough layer under the bottom layer to secure the filling in the dough pocket. Prick the top of the dough with a fork, so the pastry will vent while cooking. Brush the top with egg and bake in the middle of the oven for 30 minutes or until golden brown.

7. This lasagna-style dish goes great with a tossed salad.

Note: For reliable results, use Pepperidge Farm brand frozen pastry sheets.

Spinach Borek

Serves 12

Known in Greek cuisine as spanakopita, this spinach-stuffed pastry is as commonplace on the Armenian table as on the Greek. It's a dependable crowd pleaser.

The Filling:
1 medium-sized onion, chopped
2 tablespoons butter
2 pounds fresh spinach (about 26 cups), coarsely chopped, or
3 packages (10 ounces) frozen chopped spinach, thawed and pressed dry
3 large eggs, beaten
½ pound feta cheese, crumbled (about 1½ cups)
¼ cup chopped fresh flat-leaf parsley
2 tablespoons snipped fresh dill
1 teaspoon salt
¼ teaspoon ground black pepper

The Shell:
⅜ pound (1½ sticks) butter, melted
1 package phyllo dough (see Glossary, page 284)

1. In a large deep-sided skillet, sauté the onion in butter over medium heat until tender, about 10 minutes. Add the spinach, cover, and cook for 2 minutes, or until wilted. Remove from heat and spoon into a large mixing bowl.
2. In a smaller mixing bowl, combine the eggs, cheese, parsley, dill, salt, and pepper. Mix well. Pour over the spinach and toss.
3. Preheat the oven to 350 degrees. Remove the phyllo dough from its packaging. Cover immediately with 2 overlapping sheets of plastic wrap and a clean, slightly moistened kitchen towel to prevent the dough from drying before use.
4. Brush the bottom of the baking tray with melted butter. Layer 10 sheets of phyllo dough on top of one another, brushing each with melted butter

as it is laid. Spread the filling evenly over the top. Cover with the remaining 10 sheets of dough, buttering and layering each sheet as before.

5. Pour any remaining butter over the top, then cut the stuffed pastry with a sharp knife into 12 rectangular pieces. If freezing, wrap the tray well with plastic wrap, cover with tin foil, and freeze until ready to bake.

6. If baking, place in the middle of the oven and bake for 30 minutes, or until top is golden brown. (If the tray has been frozen, thaw completely before baking.)

7. Serve as a side dish or as a meal with salad.

Chicken and Spinach Borek

Makes 12

This chicken-stuffed phyllo dish is a playful invention of mine that errs on the rich side. Serve with a tossed green salad for a gratifying lunch or dinner.

The Filling:
1 onion, chopped
2 tablespoons olive oil
10 ounces fresh spinach (about 8 cups), coarsely chopped, or
1 package (10 ounces) frozen chopped spinach, thawed and pressed dry
3 boneless, skinless breasts of chicken, cut into 1-inch cubes
1 tablespoon butter
1 teaspoon salt
½ teaspoon ground black pepper
½ pound feta cheese, crumbled (about 1½ cups)
1 large egg, beaten slightly

The Shell:
1 package phyllo dough (see Glossary, page 284)
⅜ pound (1½ sticks) butter, melted

1. In a large deep-sided skillet, gently cook the onion in the olive oil over moderate heat, stirring occasionally, until tender, about 10 minutes.
2. Lower heat and add the spinach. Cover and cook for about 2 minutes. Remove from heat and transfer to a large mixing bowl.
3. In the same skillet, cook the chicken chunks in the butter, salt, and pepper over a medium-low heat, stirring frequently, until the pink of the meat just disappears. Remove from heat and transfer to a cutting board. Allow the chicken to cool slightly before chopping it into smaller pieces. Add to the spinach, tossing to mix.
4. In a small bowl, mix the crumbled feta with the egg, then add it to the chicken and mix well.
5. Preheat the oven to 350 degrees. Remove the phyllo dough from its packaging. Cover immediately with 2 overlapping sheets of plastic wrap

and a clean, slightly moistened kitchen towel to prevent the dough from drying before use.

6. Brush the bottom of the baking tray with butter. Lay 1 phyllo sheet in the buttered tray. Working quickly, brush it with butter and lay a second layer of dough; repeat until you have 10 sheets in the tray.

7. Spread the chicken mixture evenly over the phyllo and layer the remaining 10 sheets of dough on top, buttering between each sheet as before. Brush the top with butter and, with a sharp knife, cut into 12 individual serving-size squares.

8. Bake in the middle of the oven for about 25 minutes, or until the top is golden brown.

9. Serve warm with a tossed salad.

Note: For a slightly different flavor, add a few teaspoons of snipped fresh dill to the filling. For a different look, follow the instructions on page 124 to fold triangles.

Summer Squash and Zucchini Borek

Serves 12

When squash is disguised in a pie, my family asks for seconds. A miracle really . . . since summer squash and zucchini are two vegetables that, in my house, tend not to be eaten when prepared any other way.

The Filling:
4 medium yellow summer squash, coarsely shredded (about 4 cups)
4 medium zucchini, coarsely shredded (about 4 cups)
½ teaspoon salt
1 large onion, finely chopped
1 tablespoon butter
3 large eggs, slightly beaten
1 bunch fresh flat-leaf parsley, chopped
2 tablespoons snipped fresh dill
¼ teaspoon ground black pepper
½ pound feta cheese, crumbled (about 1½ cups)

The Shell:
1 package phyllo dough (see Glossary, page 284), or substitute
Pepperidge Farm brand frozen pastry sheets rolled out to fit
a 12 x 17 x 1-inch baking tray on a floured work-surface
⅜ pound (1½ sticks) butter, melted if using phyllo, or
¼ pound (1 stick) butter, melted if using pastry sheets
1 large egg, beaten (egg wash is used with pastry sheets only)

1. In a large mixing bowl, combine the shredded squash and zucchini. Sprinkle with the salt. Let stand for 15 minutes. The squashes will sweat.
2. Meanwhile, place the chopped onion and butter in a skillet and cook over medium heat until the onions are tender, about 10 minutes. Remove from heat and set aside.
3. Transfer the squash, handfuls at a time, to a fine-webbed strainer and squeeze out all excess juice. Place the squeezed squash in a large clean bowl and mix in the cooked onion.

4. In a smaller mixing bowl combine the eggs, parsley, dill, pepper, and feta cheese. Add this mixture to the squash and toss until well mixed.

5. Preheat the oven to 350 degrees. If using phyllo, remove from its packaging. Cover immediately with 2 overlapping sheets of plastic wrap and a clean, slightly moistened kitchen towel to prevent the dough from drying before use.

6. Brush the baking tray with butter and layer 10 sheets of phyllo dough in it, buttering each phyllo sheet as it is laid. (If using pastry sheets, place one sheet in the buttered tray.)

7. Pour off all excess juices from the filling mixture before spreading it evenly over the dough. This is important! If you leave too much moisture in the squash, the bottom dough layer will be soggy.

8. Cover the stuffing with the remaining sheets of phyllo, making sure to butter each sheet and the top sheet. With a sharp knife, cut through the phyllo, making 12 squares. (If using pastry sheets, place the second sheet over the squash mixture, fold the edges under, and crimp to secure the pastry pocket closed. With a sharp knife, cut slits in the top to allow the borek to vent while cooking. Brush the top with egg wash.)

9. Bake immediately for 30 minutes or until brown on top.

10. Serve warm. This borek complements any meat dish.

Spiced Lamb Pies

Serves 8

The Filling:
1 medium-sized onion, finely chopped
1 tablespoon butter
1 pound ground lamb
1 can (14½ ounces) peeled, diced tomatoes, drained
½ teaspoon salt
¼ teaspoon ground black pepper
¼ teaspoon Baharat Spice (page 137)
1 bunch fresh flat-leaf parsley, chopped
2 tablespoons chopped Toasted Pine Nuts (page 43)

The Shell:
1 package (2 sheets) frozen puff pastry sheet dough, thawed (for best
results, use Pepperidge Farm brand frozen pastry sheets)
White all-purpose flour for rolling
1 large egg, slightly beaten

Special Equipment:
2 (9-inch) pie plates
Heavy rolling pin

1. In a large deep-sided skillet, sauté the onions in the butter over moderate heat until tender, about 10 minutes. Add the lamb, breaking it into pea-sized pieces with a fork. Cook, stirring frequently, until the meat is no longer pink.
2. Remove from heat and drain excess fat. Return the skillet to the heat and add the tomatoes, salt, pepper, and baharat spice. Mix well and simmer for 10 minutes or until the mixture is almost dry.
3. Remove from heat. Add the parsley and pine nuts. Toss to mix and set aside to cool while rolling out the dough.
4. Preheat the oven to 350 degrees.

5. Remove the thawed pastry sheets from the package. Cut each sheet approximately in half—with one piece slightly larger than the other. On a well-floured work surface, roll the larger piece into a thin sheet that covers the bottom of the pie plate. Lay the dough in the plate. Spoon half of the meat mixture evenly over the dough. Roll out the second, smaller piece of dough and cover the meat with it. Cut the edge of the dough to fit, then crimp the edges together. Repeat with the other pastry sheet, assembling a second 9-inch pie.

6. Brush the top of each pie with beaten egg and cut a few slits in each top with a sharp knife so the pies will vent as they cook. Bake the pies in the center of the oven for about 18 minutes or until golden on top.

7. Serve hot with tossed greens for a appetizing luncheon treat.

Baharat Spice

2 tablespoons ground black pepper
1 tablespoons ground coriander seeds
1 tablespoon ground cinnamon
1 tablespoon ground cloves
1½ tablespoons ground cumin
½ teaspoon cardamom
1 tablespoon ground nutmeg
2 tablespoons paprika

1. Mix all ingredients together in a bowl.
2. Store in an airtight container.

Note: You can buy this spice premixed at gourmet stores. Or substitute Garam Masala; it's basically the same mix.

Scallion and Feta Cheese Pie

Serves 10

The Shell (see Note):
2½ cups white all-purpose flour, plus additional for rolling
½ teaspoon salt
¼ pound (1 stick) butter, firm
1 egg yolk, slightly beaten
⅓ cup cold water

The Filling:
5 - 6 scallion bundles (6 - 7 in a bundle)
¼ cup olive oil
½ pound feta cheese, crumbled (about 1½ cups)
1 large bunch fresh flat-leaf parsley, finely chopped
½ teaspoon ground black pepper
4 large eggs, beaten
1 teaspoon milk

Special Equipment:
1 (9-inch deep-sided) pie plate
Heavy rolling pin

1. Prepare the dough by sifting the flour and salt into a mixing bowl. Cut the butter into small pieces. Use a large fork to rub the butter into the flour until the mixture resembles fine crumbs.
2. Add the slightly beaten yolk and water. Knead to a soft, smooth dough. Cover and leave the dough to rest for 20 to 30 minutes.
3. Make the filling by first finely dicing the white and tender green sections of the scallions, about 2 cups. Combine the diced scallions and olive oil in a skillet and simmer over moderate heat until tender, about 10 minutes. Transfer the cooked scallions to a large mixing bowl. Add the cheese, parsley, and pepper, tossing to mix.
4. Beat the eggs in a separate bowl. Set 2 teaspoons of egg aside and add the remainder to the scallion mixture. Blend the ingredients together well.

5. Preheat the oven to 400 degrees.
6. To assemble the pie, divide the pastry in 2 pieces, 1 slightly larger than the other. Roll out the larger piece on a floured work surface. Lay it in the pie plate. Spread the scallion filling on top. Roll out the remaining dough and place it over the filling. Crimp the top and bottom pastry layers together, brushing with water, if necessary, to help it stick.
7. Add the milk to the reserved egg. Whip with a fork until frothy, then brush over the top of the pie. Cut slits in the top crust with a knife. Bake in the center of the oven for 30 minutes or until golden brown on top. Let stand for 10 minutes before cutting into individual serving slices.
8. Serve with a tossed green salad.

Note: Substituting frozen pie crust or preparing crust from a mix works, too.

MAIN COURSES

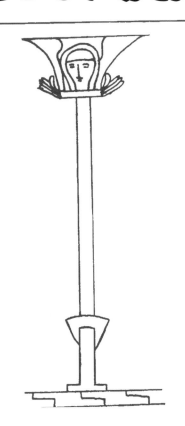

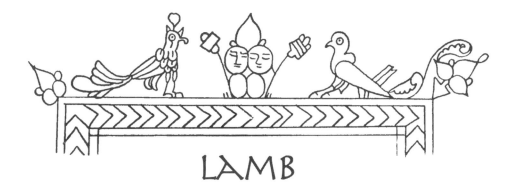

LAMB

Shish Kebab

Serves 8

Across the United States, Armenian picnics are held on Sunday afternoons beginning in late June. Today, most picnics are church fund-raisers held on church grounds, but when I was young, my extended family of aunts, uncles, and cousins would gather at my grandparents' house after church, pile into the family cars, and head to the picnic grounds out in the country.

I remember I could hardly wait for my father to park the car in the field-turned-parking-lot for the day; I was so excited. Guided by the beat of the dumbeg (a drum-like instrument) and the smell of roasting lamb, my cousins and I would jump out of the car and race to the picnic area, where we'd see lines of dancers weaving across the open-air dance floor and tables of people talking, smoking, drinking coffee, and playing backgammon. The women gossiped. The men argued politics. The kids played tag, darted between dancers with linked pinky fingers, or explored the nearby frog pond. Then we all ate skewered grilled lamb chunks on plates heaped high with rice pilaf, tossed green salad, and soft, thick pita bread.

Shish kebab dates back very far and seems to have originated with the mountain folk of the Caucasus, who, during their migrations, skewered game with their sword blades and roasted it over the fire. Here is my picnic-styled version of this signature feast.

3½ - 4 pounds leg of lamb, de-boned, trimmed of fat and gristle,
and cut into 1½-inch cubes

The Marinade:
2 onions, quartered
3 cloves of garlic, coarsely chopped
¼ cup chopped fresh flat-leaf parsley
2 - 3 tablespoons olive oil
1 tablespoon balsamic or red wine vinegar
1 tablespoon salt
½ teaspoon ground black pepper
½ teaspoon cayenne

Vegetables:
4 red onions, quartered
4 Italian peppers
24 cherry tomatoes

Special Equipment:
Wooden skewers, soaked 1 hour in cold water, or metal skewers

1. Place the lamb cubes in a large mixing bowl or plastic container.
2. Combine the marinade ingredients, mixing well, and pour over the lamb; toss to coat. Cover and refrigerate for at least 8 hours (overnight).
3. Light the grill. When the fire is medium-hot, place the onions and peppers directly on the lightly oiled grill rack. Cook, turning frequently, until the onions darken and the pepper skins blister. Remove from the heat to cool; peel, remove seeds, and pull into strips. Serve the onions and peppers together on a dish.
4. Skewer the tomatoes. Set aside.
5. Skewer the marinated lamb cubes and grill them directly on the lightly oiled rack over a moderately hot fire, turning once, until crispy outside and medium pink inside, about 8 minutes.
6. When the meat is almost done, place the tomato skewers on the grill and cook, turning, until the tomato skins begin to split and the flesh wilts, about 4 minutes.

7. Transfer the grilled meat and tomatoes to a large mixing bowl. Toss to mix. Serve on a large serving platter with pilaf, the roasted onions and peppers, a tossed green salad, and pita bread alongside.

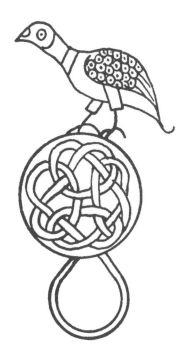

Lamb Chops on the Grill

Serves 4 to 6

Armenians are passionate about grilled lamb. In my experience, nothing comes close to the pleasure of eating a hunk of freshly roasted lamb, dripping with hot fat right off the spit, by an open fire in the Caucasian mountains. Alas, we live in the United States where lamb chops are naturally lean and a little bit expensive. For me, their ease of preparation plus their rich flavor, combined with a quick walk down memory lane, transports me right back to an Armenian mountainside campfire ringed with friends.

The Marinade (optional):
Juice of 3 lemons
2 large cloves garlic, crushed
½ teaspoon ground black pepper

6 lamb chops

1. In a small mixing bowl, whisk together lemon juice, garlic, and pepper.
2. Place the lamb chops in a container. Pour in marinade, cover, and place in the refrigerator for at least 2 hours, turning chops at least once.
3. Or forget the marinade, fire up the grill, throw the chops on a slightly greased rack over a hot flame, and cook until slightly pink in the center, about 5 minutes a side.
4. Serve with pilaf, grilled eggplant, and a tossed green salad for the perfect summertime meal.

Roast Leg of Lamb

Serves 8

I use this simple, no-frills recipe to prepare my lamb. The salt locks the juice into the meat—which comes out tender and moist.

6½- to 7-pound leg of lamb
3 cloves garlic, peeled and cut lengthwise into slivers
1 teaspoon oregano
2 teaspoons salt
½ teaspoon ground black pepper
Juice of 2 lemons

1. Preheat the oven to 450 degrees.
2. With the tip of a small, sharp knife, slice ¼-inch deep incisions on the fat side of the lamb and insert a sliver of garlic into each cut. Distribute the garlic evenly.
3. Combine the oregano, salt, and black pepper in a small bowl and press the mixture firmly all over the surface of the lamb.
4. Place the leg, fat side up, on a rack in a shallow roasting pan and roast it uncovered in the middle of the oven for 20 minutes.
5. Reduce the oven temperature to 350 degrees. Baste the leg with lemon juice and continue basting periodically with the remaining lemon juice while roasting the lamb for another 1 to 1½ hours depending on taste. It's best if you trust the roasting times and don't cut into the leg until near the end of the suggested time. If you prefer to use a meat thermometer, use the following temperatures as a guide: 140° for rare, 150° for medium, and 160° for well done.
6. Let roast rest for 10 minutes before carving. Complement the simple, rich flavor of lamb with a side of pilaf and a medley of grilled vegetables.

Note: If roasting the leg of lamb on an outside grill, place the leg directly on a lightly oiled grill rack, cover, and cook until done.

Izmir Kufteh

Serves 8

Lean, spicy lamb meatballs afloat in a light onion and tomato sauce—Izmir kufteh is an Armenian dish worthy of its namesake. Situated across the Aegean Sea from Greece, Izmir, also known as Smyrna, is one of the oldest cities of the Mediterranean world. It is the alleged birthplace of Homer and one of the earliest seats of Christianity. The port was home to a large European population until 1922, when Turkish forces set it on fire and its Christian population fled. Politics aside, you can see and taste the influence of both Greek and Italian cuisine on this special dish. Served with bulgur pilaf and a tossed green salad, Izmir kufteh is a rare culinary delight.

The Meatballs:
2 pounds very lean (95% lean) ground lamb (kheyma meat)
3 cloves of garlic, pressed
1 teaspoon salt
¾ teaspoon ground black pepper
½ teaspoon cayenne
2 eggs, slightly beaten
1 cup plain bread crumbs
½ teaspoon Baharat Spice (page 137), or substitute ¼ teaspoon allspice,
⅛ teaspoon ground cloves, ⅛ teaspoon cayenne, and pinches of ground cinnamon and nutmeg
Vegetable oil

The Sauce:
4 tablespoons (½ stick) butter
1 onion, sliced thin in semicircles
½ teaspoon salt
¼ cup finely chopped fresh flat-leaf parsley
2 cans (14½ ounces) peeled, diced tomatoes
Pinch of ground cinnamon

1. Mix the meat, garlic, salt, black pepper, cayenne, eggs, bread crumbs, and baharat spice in a large bowl. Shape the meat mixture into little hamburgers, about 1½-inches in diameter.

2. Heat 1-inch-deep vegetable oil in a large, deep-sided skillet until hot. Fry the patties in the hot oil until browned, about 3 minutes total, flipping once. The patties will puff up into egg-shaped pieces called kuftehs. Drain the kuftehs on paper towels to remove excess oil.

3. Melt the butter in a second large deep-sided skillet, add the onion slices, and cook over medium heat, stirring occasionally, until onions soften, about 10 minutes. Add the salt, parsley, tomato, cinnamon, and the kuftehs. Cover and simmer for about 10 minutes.

4. Spoon over pilaf and serve with a salad for a complete meal.

Armenian Tartare

Kheyma

Serves 4

Saturday nights at Grandma's house meant kheyma when I was growing up. I remember watching her grind her own meat (three times!) through a meat grinder she would clamp to the edge of her kitchen sink. I still have that grinder in my basement. Thankfully, a reputable butcher handles that arduous task today.

If your budget allows, substitute lamb for beef. If handled properly and kept well refrigerated, raw lamb is safer to eat and tastier, too. Do not eat this dish if you are or think you may be pregnant. There is a remote possibility of acquiring toxoplasmosis from the raw meat. Do not eat it if you have any concern about eating raw meat. In fact, I don't expect anyone who hasn't been weaned on this dish to try it, but for those of us who were—my grandma's kheyma was the best!

½ cup fine-grain bulgur
1 small onion, finely chopped
1 teaspoon cayenne
1 - 1½ teaspoons salt
½ teaspoon ground cumin
⅛ teaspoon ground cinnamon
1 pound beef or lamb kheyma meat
Ice cubes, if necessary

The Toppings:
1 large bunch fresh flat-leaf parsley, chopped
1 large onion, chopped

1. Place the bulgur in a large bowl and add enough cold water to cover it about ¼-inch. Stir and let stand 20 minutes, or until the grain soaks up all of the water.

2. Stir the onion, cayenne, salt, cumin, and cinnamon into the bulgur.

3. Wash your hands thoroughly in hot, soapy water and rinse well. Add the meat and knead as if making bread, until the bulgur and meat are blended. If the mixture seems too dry, add ice cubes, 1 or 2 at a time, as you knead.

3. Form the meat into balls about 2-inches in diameter. Set on a serving plate and garnish with fresh chopped parsley and onions.

4. Serve immediately with a fresh tossed green salad and Armenian Cracker Bread (page 189) or pita.

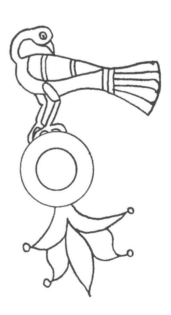

Harpout Kufteh

Makes about 2 dozen

Harpout or kharpert, meaning "stone fortress," was an Armenian-inhabited town in the Ottoman Empire, renowned for its cooking. Legend has it that, in 1914, just before Turkish gendarmes deported one woman from her village, she stuffed her last batch of kuftehs with gold coins. Her culinary ingenuity saved her life, because the hidden money bought her enough advantages on the march into the desert that she survived.

The Stuffing:
½ pound ground lamb (80% lean)
1 large onion, finely chopped
¼ teaspoon allspice
¼ teaspoon ground clove
½ teaspoon salt
¼ teaspoon ground black pepper
⅓ cup finely chopped fresh flat-leaf parsley

The Crust:
3 cups fine-grain bulgur
1 pound very lean (95% lean) ground lamb (kheyma meat)
½ teaspoon salt
¼ teaspoon ground black pepper

The Broth:
8 cups chicken broth

1. To prepare the stuffing, sauté the lamb, onion, allspice, clove, salt, and pepper in a large skillet over low heat, stirring occasionally, until the meat is evenly browned and the onion soft. Remove from heat and stir in the fresh parsley. Cool to room temperature. (The stuffing can be made a few days ahead of time and kept refrigerated in an airtight container until ready to use.)

2. Prepare the meatball crust by placing the bulgur in a mixing bowl, adding cold water, and stirring a couple of times, until the grain is covered. Let stand 10 minutes, or until most of the water is absorbed.

3. In a larger mixing bowl, combine the very lean (kheyma) meat with the soaked bulgur. Knead in the salt and pepper. Knead by hand until the meat is smooth and elastic, like bread dough. If the mixture is dry and crumbly, add very cold water, a tablespoon at a time.

4. Once you are satisfied with the texture, roll small sections into walnut-sized balls. Make a hole in the center of each ball with your fingers, and fill the hole with a teaspoon of cooled stuffing. Gently close the hole by pushing the outer crust around the hole. Sometimes it helps to dip your fingers in cold water before kneading the hole closed.

5. Pour the chicken broth into a large pot and bring it to a boil over high heat. Add the stuffed meatballs, now called kuftehs, a few at a time. At first the kuftehs will sink to the bottom, but when cooked they should rise to the surface and float. This will take about 8 minutes. With a slotted spoon, remove the kuftehs to a large serving bowl and reserve the broth for Yogurt Soup with Harpout Kuftehs (page 121).

6. Boiled kuftehs never make it to the soup stage in my family, at least not with my brother around. Boiled kuftehs are his all-time favorite food. His preferred method of consumption is to grab one from of the bowl as they are cooling and wolf it down in a few bites. If you can, rescue a dozen or so and try the soup recipe.

Baked Stuffed Meat Pie

Sini Kufteh

Serves 10

Americans best conceptualize this dish as a thin meatloaf-like sheet, while Armenians think of it as a flattened kufteh. Many Middle Eastern food writers will refer to it as a kibbeh (an Arabic term) or sini kufteh (the Turkish name). Semantics aside, this one-pan dish is a spiced center of ground lamb and onions in a crust of bulgur and lean ground meat. It's easy to make and delicious to eat, and one baking tray will generously feed a small army of guests.

The Filling:
3 onions, finely chopped
1 tablespoon butter
1 pound ground lamb (80% lean)
1 large bunch fresh flat-leaf parsley, finely chopped
1½ teaspoons salt
½ teaspoon cayenne
½ teaspoon ground cumin
¼ teaspoon allspice
½ cup chopped Toasted Pine Nuts (page 43)

The Crust:
1½ cups fine-grain bulgur
1 pound very lean (at least 90% lean) ground lamb (kheyma meat)
1½ teaspoons ground black pepper
1½ teaspoons salt
Solid shortening (about ½ cup)

The Topping:
Plain yogurt (optional)

Special Equipment:
1 (12 x 17 x 1-inch) baking sheet, greased with solid shortening
and set aside

1. To make the filling, cook the onions in a large skillet with the butter over medium heat, stirring occasionally, until tender and translucent, about 10 minutes. Add the lamb and cook, stirring and breaking up lumps, until the meat is no longer pink. Remove from heat and pour off excess fat. Stir in the parsley, spices, and nuts. Set aside.

2. To prepare the crust, place the bulgur in a mixing bowl and add enough cold water to cover it about 1 inch. Stir and let sit for 10 minutes. Most of the water will be absorbed. Pour off excess, then transfer the wet bulgur to a larger mixing bowl and add the lamb, salt, and pepper. Knead until smooth and well mixed, moistening your hands with cold water, if necessary. Divide into two equal parts.

3. Preheat the oven to 375 degrees.

4. Assemble the pie. The key to this dish is the crust—the thinner the better. Press half of the crust mixture onto the bottom of the prepared baking sheet. Gently pat the filling evenly on top. Cover the filling with the remaining crust mixture. The easiest way to do this is to roll small balls of meat in your hands then flatten each ball with your palms. Lay flattened meat over the filling until it completely covers the top of the baking sheet.

5. Smooth the top of the pie by moistening your hands with water and smoothing the crust with them. With a knife, cut the sheet into serving-sized diamonds. Finally, dab the solid shortening in teaspoon-sized clumps over the top, spacing the clumps 2½-inches apart. (It may seem like you are using a sinful amount of shortening, but fight any urge to skimp; otherwise your pie will be dry.)

6. Bake for about 45 minutes or until the meat is browned through.

7. Remove from the oven and preheat the broiler. Broil the pie 6 inches from the heat until the top is golden brown and crusty, about 3 to 5 minutes. Let stand 5 minutes before serving.

8. Serve topped with a dollop of yogurt.

Grilled Lamb Patties

Losh Kebabs

Serves 8

Kick off the summer barbecue season with these spiced lamb patties Armenians call losh kebabs.

1 tablespoon butter
1 small onion, finely chopped
1 pound ground lamb
¾ cup fine-grain bulgur
1 can (14½ ounces) peeled, diced tomatoes
¼ cup chopped fresh flat-leaf parsley
½ teaspoon ground cumin
1 teaspoon salt
¼ teaspoon ground black pepper
1 teaspoon finely chopped fresh mint, or ¼ teaspoon dried mint (optional)
1 cup Yogurt Sauce (page 226) (optional)

1. In a skillet, sauté the onion in the butter over moderate heat until the onion softens and turns golden, about 10 minutes. Transfer to a large mixing bowl.
2. Add the lamb, bulgur, tomatoes, parsley, spices, and mint, if desired. Knead the meat until the ingredients are evenly mixed. Lamb has a tendency to get tough when over-handled, so take care not to over-knead.
3. Let rest for about 10 minutes before shaping the meat into patties. This allows the bulgur to soften by soaking up the juices.
4. Prepare the grill for cooking. Grill the patties over high heat until crusty outside and moist and tender inside, about 5 minutes per side.
5. For a real treat, serve these patties in a pita round, topped with a thick juicy slice of fresh tomato and drizzled with Yogurt Sauce. Yum, yum.

Note: These lamb burgers can be cooked on the stovetop or broiled. The cooking time is about the same.

Fried Stuffed Zucchini

Serves 8

Few dishes offer the delicate mix of flavors that stuffed vegetables (dolmas) offer, nor is the inherent thrift of the cuisine as apparent. When made together, Fried Stuffed Zucchini and Fried Zucchini Pancakes (page 78) leave no part of the garden-fresh squash unused.

10 (8-inch long) zucchini
1 pound ground lamb
1 onion, finely chopped
¼ cup chopped fresh flat-leaf parsley
1 teaspoon salt
½ teaspoon ground black pepper
¼ teaspoon cayenne
Vegetable oil
1 can (14½ ounces) peeled, diced tomatoes

1. Cut each zucchini in half. Trim the stems. With a small coring knife, core each squash half until the sides are about ⅛-inch thick. Transfer the squash pulp into a saucepan and use to prepare Fried Zucchini Pancakes (page 78). Set hollowed zucchinis aside.
2. Combine the meat, onion, parsley, salt, and peppers in a bowl. Stuff the hollowed squashes with meat mixture.
3. In a deep-sided skillet, heat ¼-inch of oil over moderately high heat until hot but not smoking. Then fry the stuffed squash in the very hot oil. Turn them until the skins darken evenly on all sides, about 10 minutes. When done, remove and drain on paper towels.
4. Preheat the oven to 350 degrees.
5. Arrange the fried stuffed squash in a baking dish. Pour the tomatoes on top, cover, and bake for 45 minutes.
6. Serve with pilaf and yogurt.

Stuffed Pepper Dolmas

Serves 6

For those brought up thinking that meat and vegetables are cooked separately, meeting for the first time on the dinner plate, stuffed vegetables (called dolmas) present a major departure from the norm. But the early marriage of meat and vegetable during preparation is commonplace in Middle Eastern cuisine.

This recipe is my personal favorite. Stuffed Italian peppers offer an inexpensive, easy-to-make, low-fat, nutritious, and delicious everyday meal. In my home, we eat these dolmas as often as the average family eats pizza!

8 Italian peppers (see Note)
1 pound ground lamb
½ cup short-grain rice
½ onion, finely chopped
½ cup chopped fresh flat-leaf parsley
1 teaspoon salt
¼ teaspoon ground black pepper
1 can (14½ ounces) peeled, diced tomatoes
Juice of 1 lemon
½ teaspoon dried mint
Plain yogurt (optional)

1. Wash the peppers. Cut tops off and remove seeds. Set aside.
2. Mix the meat, rice, onion, parsley, salt, and half of the can of tomatoes in a large mixing bowl.
3. Stuff the cored peppers with meat.
4. Arrange the stuffed peppers in a large pot. Pour the remaining tomatoes over the top. Add the lemon juice, mint, and a little water, so that there is approximately 1-inch of liquid in the bottom of the pan.
5. Cover and bring to a boil. Lower the heat and simmer, covered, for about 45 minutes, or until the peppers are tender.
6. Serve topped with a dollop of yogurt and accompany with pita bread.

Note: Substitute bell peppers, small zucchinis, small eggplants, tomatoes, grape leaves, or blanched cabbage leaves for the Italian peppers. Almost any vegetable can be stuffed and boiled.

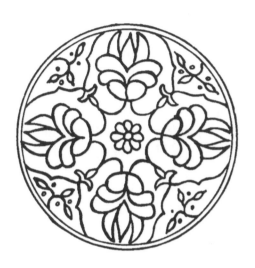

Lamb-Stuffed Grape Leaves

Sarma

Serves 4

The Stuffing:
1 pound ground lamb
½ cup coarse-grain bulgur or short-grain rice
1 small onion, finely chopped
½ cup chopped fresh flat-leaf parsley
1 teaspoon salt
¼ teaspoon ground black pepper
¼ teaspoon cayenne
⅓ cup tomato paste
1 cup water
Juice of 1 lemon

25 large grape leaves, plus a few to line the pot
Plain yogurt

1. Combine the stuffing ingredients in a large mixing bowl.
2. If using store-bought grape leaves, rinse them several times in water, draining each time. If using fresh frozen grape leaves (page 28), plunge leaves in boiling salted water until the color darkens to olive, about 1 minute. Remove immediately, rinse with cold water, and drain.
3. Taking 1 leaf at a time, place the back of the leaf on a flat work surface in front of you. Spoon about a tablespoon of filling onto the middle of the leaf and fold the bottom portion of the leaf over the stuffing. Fold the sides in. Finish by rolling the leaf up, away from you on the work surface, so that the stuffed leaf resembles a small hot dog. Line a large pot with extra leaves, and place the tightly rolled leaf in the pot. Repeat until all leaves are stuffed and arranged.
4. Place a dinner plate, bottom-side up, over the stuffed leaves to secure them, and add enough water to cover. Quickly bring the pot to a boil, turn the heat lower, cover, and simmer for 30 minutes.

5. Serve hot, garnished with a dollop of yogurt.

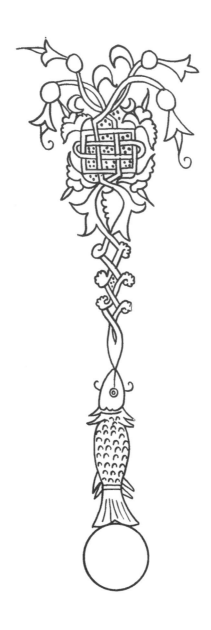

Cabbage Rolls

Lahana Dolma

Serves 8

Cabbage is a vegetable flattered by every method of cooking. Flash-cooked, well-cooked, or over-cooked, it's always deliciously sweet. Prepare this dish with confidence. You can't ruin it.

1 large head of cabbage
Salt

The Stuffing:
1 medium onion, finely chopped
2 tablespoons olive oil
1 pound ground lamb
1 cup short-grain rice
¼ teaspoon allspice
½ teaspoon salt
¼ teaspoon ground black pepper
¼ cup water

To Finish:
4 cloves garlic, chopped
Salt
Juice of 2 lemons
1 teaspoon dried mint
Plain yogurt

1. Core the cabbage and remove all leaves. Fill a pot with water and salt generously. Bring the water to a boil and boil the leaves until limp, about 1 minute. Drain the boiled leaves in a colander and let cool.
2. Cut the larger leaves in half, removing the rib. For smaller leaves, just cut out the thicker part of the rib. Line a pot with ribs and any torn leaves.

3. Gently sauté the onions in olive oil in a deep-sided skillet over medium heat until soft, about 10 minutes.

4. Combine the cooked onions with the lamb in a mixing bowl. Add the remaining stuffing ingredients and mix well.

5. Arrange 1 leaf at a time, back side up, on a flat work surface in front of you. Place a tablespoon of filling at the bottom edge of the leaf, tuck in both sides, and roll the leaf like a sausage.

6. Closely pack the rolls, flap side down, together in the lined pot.

7. Combine the garlic, salt, lemon juice, and mint in a mixing bowl. Add enough water so that, when poured over the rolls, the liquid just covers the stuffed leaves.

8. Place a dinner plate, bottom-side up, on top of the rolls to secure them. Cover the pan and bring to a boil quickly over high heat. Turn the heat down, and simmer, covered, for 1 hour.

9. Serve hot, garnished with a dollop of yogurt.

Eggplant and Ground Lamb

Serves 8

My aunt went all out preparing her Thanksgiving meal for the family. I had to search to find this dish somewhere on the table, sandwiched between platters of roasted chicken, baked ham, boiled kufteh, bowls of pilaf, turnips, mashed potatoes, gravy, and a minimum of two salads. But I always found it, because for me one serving of this casserole next to a heaping pile of pilaf was enough to satisfy my holiday appetite.

I don't wait for a holiday to make this dish. It's a once-a-week favorite in my home, and the best part is, a few days in the refrigerator ripens the flavors and makes it even better.

1 medium eggplant, peeled
Salt
¼ cup olive oil
2 small cloves garlic, minced
1 medium onion, chopped
1 green pepper, finely chopped
1 pound ground lamb
1 teaspoon salt
½ teaspoon ground black pepper
¼ teaspoon cayenne
1 can (14½ ounces) peeled, diced tomatoes
¼ cup finely chopped fresh flat-leaf parsley

1. Slice the eggplant into rounds, about ¼-inch thick. Soak the rounds in a large bowl of cold, heavily salted water for at least 20 minutes. Drain and pat slices dry with paper towels.
2. Preheat the oven to 350 degrees.
3. Brush the eggplant slices on both sides with olive oil and arrange the oiled rounds on a baking sheet. Bake for 20 minutes, then turn the slices over and bake for an additional 15 minutes, or until the eggplant is very soft. Remove from the oven and set aside to cool.

4. While the eggplant is baking, sauté the garlic and onion in the remaining olive oil over medium heat in a large deep-sided skillet until the onion is tender and translucent, about 10 minutes. Add the green pepper. Cook, stirring occasionally, for another 15 to 20 minutes, until the pepper begins to soften. Break the lamb up into the skillet and cook, stirring occasionally, until pink disappears. Stir in the salt, black pepper, cayenne, tomatoes, and parsley. Simmer, uncovered, about 15 minutes.
5. Cover the bottom of a casserole dish with meat sauce. Place a layer of eggplant over the sauce. Continue layering sauce and eggplant until both are used. Cover and bake 45 minutes, or until eggplant is mushy.
6. Serve hot, accompanied with a pilaf and cracker or pita bread.

Artichokes Stuffed with Ground Lamb

Serves 4

This is one of the tastiest dishes in the collection. During baking, the natural meat juices tenderize the artichoke leaves, transforming them into buttery delicacies.

4 large artichokes
Juice of 2 lemons
¾ pound ground lamb
1 medium onion, chopped
1 tablespoon chopped fresh flat-leaf parsley
1 tablespoon chopped Toasted Pine Nuts (page 43)
¼ teaspoon ground cumin
½ teaspoon salt
¼ teaspoon ground black pepper
1 large egg
1 medium-sized tomato, sliced into 4 slices
2 cups water

1. Cut off artichoke tops, leaving two-thirds of the heart and bottom. Scoop out inside leaves and fuzzy choke. Immediately squeeze juice from 1 of the lemons into the empty artichoke to prevent discoloring.
2. Preheat the oven to 350 degrees.
3. In a large skillet, fry the lamb with the onions over moderate heat until the meat is browned and the onions tender, about 10 minutes.
4. Stir in the parsley, pine nuts, cumin, salt, and pepper.
5. Transfer to a mixing bowl. Add the egg, mixing well. The egg will help hold the stuffing mixture together.
6. Fill the center of each artichoke with stuffing and place them in a deep-sided baking pan or casserole dish. Cover each with 1 tomato slice.
7. Once the stuffed artichokes are arranged, add the water and the juice from the remaining lemon to the pan. Cover and bake for 1½ hours.
8. Serve hot with pilaf for a complete meal.

Lamb with Quince Slices

Serves 4

The cool days of autumn and early darkness tempt our desire for comfort foods. Satisfy those desires by serving this light entrée over a pillow of pilaf for a dish filled with a subtle balance of flavors, colors, and aromas that combine the simple and the exotic. Followed by a dessert that's a little more "sinful" than average, the result is an unforgettable dining experience.

2 onions, chopped
6 tablespoons (¾ stick) butter
2-pound boneless leg of lamb, fat trimmed off and cut into 1-inch cubes
1 teaspoon salt
½ teaspoon ground black pepper
½ teaspoon ground cumin
2 cups water
2 large quinces, peeled, cored, and sliced
¼ cup fresh lemon juice (juice of about 4 lemons)
½ cup yellow split peas

1. In a large deep-sided skillet, brown the onions in 3 tablespoons butter over moderate heat, stirring occasionally, about 12 minutes. Add the lamb cubes and brown evenly, about 10 minutes. Stir in the salt, pepper, and cumin. Add water, cover, and simmer over low heat for 1 hour, stirring occasionally.
2. In a different skillet, sauté the quince slices in the remaining 3 tablespoons butter over moderate heat, stirring occasionally, until they soften, about 20 minutes. Set aside.
3. When the meat is tender, add the lemon juice, peas, and sautéed quince slices. Cover and simmer 35 minutes, or until the quince is soft.
4. Serve hot over rice pilaf.

Sautéed Lamb with Eggplant Purée

Sultan's Delight

Serves 4

Nicknamed Sultan's Delight, this is a royal dish, rich with the smoky, warm flavors of the Middle East. It looks hard to make and expensive to serve, but looks can be deceiving.

The Lamb:
1½ pounds lamb meat, trimmed of fat, and cut into 1-inch cubes
2 medium onions, finely chopped
2 tablespoons butter
¼ cup tomato paste
1¼ cups water
¼ teaspoon allspice
1 teaspoon salt
½ teaspoon ground black pepper
¼ cup chopped fresh flat-leaf parsley

The Purée:
1 large eggplant
1 tablespoon lemon juice
4 tablespoons (½ stick) butter
¼ cup while all-purpose flour
¾ cup milk
¼ cup fine-grain bulgur, soaked for 15 minutes in ½ cup cold water
½ cup kasseri cheese, shredded
½ teaspoon salt
¼ teaspoon ground black pepper

Special Equipment:
Blender or food processor

1. Place the lamb cubes and onion in a large deep-sided skillet with the butter. Cook over moderate heat, stirring frequently, until the onions are tender and the meat is browned on all sides, about 15 minutes.

2. Stir in the tomato paste and water. Add the allspice, salt, black pepper, and most of the parsley. (Set the remaining parsley aside to use as a garnish.) Cook, stirring occasionally, over medium-low heat until the sauce thickens, about 20 minutes.

3. Preheat the oven to 350 degrees or prepare a charcoal or gas grill.

4. Place the whole eggplant on a cookie sheet in the oven and bake for 20 minutes, or grill on a slightly oiled grill rack over moderate coals, until the eggplant is very soft and collapses like a deflated balloon. Remove from heat and cool. Peel the skin and purée the eggplant pulp in a blender or food processor. Add the lemon juice to prevent discoloring.

5. Melt the butter in a deep-sided, heavy-bottomed saucepan; stir in flour. Cook for about 2 minutes before adding the milk. Stir constantly until the mixture thickens and bubbles.

6. Add the eggplant purée and cook, stirring occasionally, over low heat until the mixture thickens. Add the soaked bulgur. Remove from heat. Stir in the shredded cheese and beat with a wooden spoon until smooth. Add the salt and pepper.

7. Spoon the eggplant into a serving dish, indent the center, and fill it with lamb. For a meal worthy of royalty, garnish with the reserved parsley and serve hot with savory Tabouli (page 85) and a rich Bulgur Pilaf (page 59).

Braised Lamb Shanks

Serves 6

It doesn't get any more primal than eating lamb off the bone, dripping in juices and swimming in bone marrow. Enjoy!

6 lamb shanks, trimmed of excess fat
Salt
Ground black pepper
2 tablespoons olive oil
1 large green bell pepper, cut into ½-inch pieces
2 small garlic cloves, finely chopped
⅛ teaspoon ground cinnamon
⅛ teaspoon allspice
¼ teaspoon ground black pepper
1 cup dry white wine
2 cans (14½ ounces) peeled, diced tomatoes
½ teaspoon salt

1. Preheat the oven to 350 degrees.
2. Sprinkle the shanks with salt and pepper. Heat the olive oil in a large deep-sided skillet over moderately high heat until hot but not smoking, then sear the shanks in batches, turning occasionally, about 5 minutes per batch. Transfer the browned shanks to a roasting pan just large enough to hold them in one layer.
3. In the same skillet, cook the bell pepper, garlic, cinnamon, allspice, and black pepper over moderate heat, stirring occasionally, until the garlic is golden, about 3 minutes. Add the wine and bring to a boil. Add the tomatoes and bring to a second boil, stirring occasionally. Add the salt and pour over the shanks. The liquid should come at least halfway up the sides of the meat.
4. Cover the roasting pan tightly with foil or a lid and cook in the middle of the oven until tender, about 2½ to 3 hours.
5. Serve the shanks, covered with sauce, immediately, accompanied by pilaf, Fried Eggplant with Yogurt Sauce (page 68), and pita bread.

Braised Lamb Shanks Wrapped in Eggplant

Serves 8

If primal bothers you, try this variation of basic lamb shanks wrapped in eggplant. Preparation is best if done as a 2-day affair.

The Eggplant:
2 eggplants (at least 10-inches long and 4-inches in diameter), peeled
Salt
¼ cup extra-virgin olive oil

6 lamb shanks, trimmed of excess fat

Day 1:
1. Cut each eggplant lengthwise into ⅓-inch-thick slices. Place slices in a large bowl of cold, heavily salted water, and soak for at least 20 minutes. Drain, and pat slices dry with paper towels.
2. Preheat the oven to 350 degrees.
3. Brush eggplant slices on both sides with olive oil and arrange on a baking sheet. Bake for 20 minutes in the oven. Turn over and bake for an additional 20 minutes until the eggplant is tender. Remove and cool before refrigerating them overnight.
4. Prepare the shanks according to the instructions provided earlier (page 170). Cool the shanks, uncovered, and discard bones and fatty tissue. Place the shank meat back in the roasting pan, cover, and refrigerate overnight.

Day 2:
5. Preheat the oven to 350 degrees.
6. Skim fat from the top of the meat and discard. Taking 1 eggplant slice at a time, roll a piece of lamb inside to form a bundle. Place each bundle back into the roasting pan. Repeat, until all eggplant slices are rolled and arranged in the pan. Bake, covered, for 45 minutes.
7. Serve hot. The shanks prepared this way have a mild, subtle flavor that many people prefer.

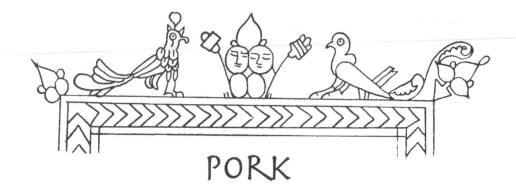

PORK

Grilled Pork Chops

Serves 4

My grandparents, and friends of their generation, never cooked or ate pork. Pork entered Armenian cuisine during Soviet times. Grilled pork chops are simple to prepare and mouth-wateringly delicious. Throw etiquette to the wind; pick the grilled chop up in your hands and gnaw the bone.

4 (1-inch-thick) pork chops with bone
Ground cumin
Salt
Ground black pepper
Cayenne (optional)
Thyme (optional)

1. Shake the cumin, salt, and black pepper, and either or both optional spices, if desired, on both sides of the chops, seasoning to taste.
2. Place the seasoned meat on the lightly oiled rack of a charcoal or gas grill over medium-hot heat. Cover and cook, about 25 minutes, turning once to brown the meat evenly on both sides.
3. Serve with pilaf and a salad.

Spiced Pork Roast

Serves 8

There is nothing quite like a pork roast when it's cold outside. This recipe is super-easy and especially delicious. Rub the roast a day or so before cooking in the special dry spice rub mixture, then pop it in the oven. The result is a flavor-packed roast that can be served with any combination of side dishes.

The Spice Rub:
1 teaspoon ground black pepper
¼ teaspoon allspice
½ teaspoon Hungarian hot paprika
½ teaspoon paprika
½ teaspoon thyme

1 (4-pound) pork roast

1. Combine the spice rub ingredients in a small bowl. Rub the spice mixture all over the raw meat. Place in an airtight plastic bag, seal, and refrigerate for a minimum of 8 hours (overnight).
2. Preheat the oven to 350 degrees.
3. Place the pork roast, fat side up, on a roasting rack in a pan. Cook in the middle of the oven for 1½ hours, or just until the last hint of pink disappears from the meat.
4. Let stand 10 minutes before serving. Try with Cumin-Glazed Carrots (page 65) and one of the potato dishes or pilaf.

Note: This spice rub is terrific on boneless turkey breast, grilled.

Roast Pork Stuffed with Shallots and Apricots

Serves 6

Stuffing pork through the center of the loin makes for a beautiful and colorful mosaic in every slice.

The Stuffing:
3 large shallots, chopped
2 tablespoons butter
3 large firm-ripe apricots, cut into ½-inch chunks, or
6 dried apricots, chopped
¼ cup chopped fresh flat-leaf parsley
½ cup plain bread crumbs
Juice of 1 lemon
½ teaspoon salt
¼ teaspoon ground black pepper

The Meat:
1 (3-pound) center cut boneless pork loin roast, not tied
Thyme
Rosemary
Salt
Ground black pepper
2 tablespoons vegetable oil

1. Make the stuffing by cooking the shallots in the butter in a large skillet, stirring occasionally, until softened, about 10 minutes. Add the apricots and cook, stirring, until slightly softened, about 3 minutes. Remove from heat and transfer to a mixing bowl. Add the parsley, bread crumbs, lemon juice, salt, and black pepper. Stir to mix.

2. Preheat the oven to 375 degrees.

3. Make a hole for the stuffing lengthwise through the pork loin by inserting a long, thin knife lengthwise from one end of the roast toward the center then repeating the cut from the opposite end. Open the incision with your fingers or the long handle of a wooden spoon to create a 1½-inch-wide

opening, then pack the channel with the stuffing, pushing from both ends toward the center.

4. Rub thyme, rosemary, salt, and black pepper over the top and bottom of the stuffed loin, to taste.

5. Heat the oil in a skillet over high heat and brown the pork on all sides, about 2 minutes. Transfer to a roasting pan. If there is any stuffing left over, spoon it over and around the roast.

6. Roast the pork loin in the middle of the oven for 1 - 1¼ hours, depending on the size of the loin. The meat should be just pink inside.

7. When done, let rest for 5 minutes. Slice and serve with pilaf and your choice of vegetables.

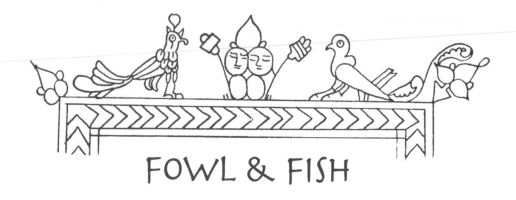

FOWL & FISH

Roasted Goose with Natural Juice Gravy

Serves 8

Cooking a goose takes time and is only done in the Armenian home kitchen in celebration of a major holiday like Christmas or New Year. It's said that there's more than one way to cook a goose. While that may be true, the Armenian way to prepare fowl follows the adage "the less you fiddle with a bird the better it'll be." Employing this method, you need to begin the preparation of this feast a few days before you are planning to serve it. But once you get the timetable down, the rest is easy.

The Bird:
1 whole (including innards) goose, 10- to 12-pounds
2 tablespoons butter, melted
1 large clove garlic, minced
Salt
Ground black pepper
6 medium onions, halved

The Gravy:
1 tablespoon cornstarch
Salt
Ground black pepper
1 tablespoon Armenian cognac (see Note)

Special Equipment:
Huge cooking pot
Fine-mesh strainer or cheesecloth

1. Most often, the goose you buy from the supermarket will be frozen. If so, defrost the bird in the refrigerator. This may take a few days, so plan ahead.

2. Because goose is a fatty bird, simmering it removes the majority of the fat and improves the crispness of the skin. Simmer the bird 1 or 2 days before your planned roasting date. Remove the neck, giblets, and wing tips from the defrosted bird. Set these aside for the gravy. Prick the skin all over with a fork.

3. Fill a jumbo-sized pot ⅔ full of water and bring to a boil over high heat. Carefully lower the bird into the boiling water, reduce the heat, and simmer gently for 45 minutes. Remove the bird and allow it to cool to room temperature before refrigerating it, uncovered, overnight.

4. Begin preparation of the gravy the same day you simmer the bird by placing the giblets and other innards, excluding the liver, in a saucepan. Add 2½ quarts of cold water and bring to a boil. Simmer uncovered for 3 hours, or until the liquid is reduced by ⅔. Strain the gravy through a fine-mesh strainer or cheesecloth. Discard the giblets because they have been cooked beyond the point of being appetizing. Cover the broth and refrigerate overnight.

5. On the day of roasting, preheat the oven to 325 degrees. Place the goose, breast side up, on a roasting rack in a roasting pan.

6. Combine the melted butter and minced garlic in a small bowl, then brush the breast, legs, and thighs of the bird with it. Salt and pepper generously. Arrange the halved onions around the goose.

7. Begin baking the goose by turning it on one side, and roasting it in the oven for 30 minutes. Then take it out of the oven, turn it onto the opposite side, return it to the oven, and roast for 30 minutes. Remove it from the oven again, turn it breast side up, return it to the oven, and roast for another 30 minutes or until the breast meat registers 150 degrees on an instant-read thermometer. Remove from the oven and let sit uncovered for 20 minutes before carving.

8. As the goose stands, continue preparing the gravy by adding 3 tablespoons of drippings from the roasting pan to a saucepan with the reserved broth. Bring the gravy to a boil and boil rapidly for about 10 minutes or until the liquid is reduced by a third. In a small bowl, mix the cornstarch with 2 tablespoons of water, then whisk into the boiling broth. Lower the heat and simmer another 5 minutes, whisking vigorously as the gravy thickens. Add salt, pepper, and cognac to taste.

9. Carve the goose. The dark, rich flavors of goose shine served alongside my savory Rice Pilaf with Pomegranate and Toasted Pine Nuts (page 62).

Note: Armenia is famous for its cognac. Imported Armenian cognac can be purchased at most liquor stores in major metropolitan areas throughout the United States. If you have to, substitute French.

Grilled Lemon Chicken

Serves 8

2 pounds skinless chicken thighs (small breasts or
legs are fine, too)

The Marinade:
Juice of 3 lemons
3 tablespoons balsamic vinegar
1 tablespoon dried mint
1 teaspoon ground cumin
1 teaspoon salt
½ teaspoon oregano
½ teaspoon thyme
¼ teaspoon ground black pepper
¼ teaspoon cayenne

1. Place the chicken in a large baking dish or plastic container.
2. Combine the marinade ingredients in a separate bowl, mixing well. Pour over the chicken, cover, and refrigerate for at least 2 hours. Turn the chicken pieces over halfway through the marinating time.
3. Prepare a charcoal or gas grill and grill the chicken over a medium-hot fire, turning as needed, until done, about 12 to 15 minutes a side.
4. For a fabulous summer meal, serve this snappy chicken with a side of pilaf, grilled eggplant, and a salad.

Boiled–Baked Rice-Stuffed Chicken

Serves 6 to 8

This recipe was one of my grandmother's specialties. By boiling a chicken stuffed with rice in a pot and then putting it in the oven to bake, she prepared a one-dish Sunday meal (minus the salad). If the "boil first—bake second" cooking process sounds unusual, it is, but so are the resulting flavors. Try this recipe on a day you are entertaining guests, not only because it's a time- and labor-saving recipe, but also because serving pilaf from the cavity of the bird is as fun as it is tasty.

1 (4-pound) whole roasting chicken

The Stuffing:
1 cup long-grain rice
1 medium onion, finely chopped
1 large bunch fresh flat-leaf parsley, finely chopped
1 tablespoon finely chopped fresh mint, or 1 teaspoon dried mint
¾ teaspoon salt
¼ teaspoon ground black pepper

Special Equipment:
Needle and thread
1 jumbo-sized pot

1. Wash the inside and outside of the chicken under cold running water. Drain, pat dry with paper towels, and set aside.
2. In a medium-sized mixing bowl, combine the stuffing ingredients.
3. Pack the cavity of the bird with stuffing. Once stuffed, thread a needle with string and sew the vent of the bird closed. You don't have to be careful or neat. Even if your chicken ends up resembling Frankenstein, don't despair, it will taste great.
4. Bring 3 quarts of water to a boil over high heat in a jumbo-sized pot. Once boiling, gently lower the stuffed chicken into the water. Reduce heat and

simmer, uncovered, for 30 minutes. The chicken will puff up like a blowfish as the pilaf stuffing cooks.

5. Preheat the oven to 350 degrees.

6. Remove the boiled chicken from the pot and place it, breast side up, in a roasting pan. Cool the cooking liquid to room temperature. Retain the broth in the refrigerator or the freezer for one of the many chicken-broth–based soups in this collection.

7. Bake the chicken, uncovered, in a baking pan set on the middle rack of the oven for about 1 hour.

8. Remove to a serving platter. Allow the bird to cool for at least 5 minutes before carving. Cut the vent string open with scissors and serve the stuffing directly from the cavity of the bird with a large serving spoon.

9. Complement the poultry and pilaf with dark-leafed tossed greens dressed with zesty Balsamic Vinaigrette (page 224) and enjoy a mini holiday feast.

✑ Swordfish Kebabs with Grilled Eggplant ✑

Serves 2 to 3

My ancestors, like most Armenian families, lived in villages located in the interior of the Ottoman Empire, far from the Mediterranean or Black Sea. Saltwater fish was virtually unknown to them. This recipe, adapted from the classic skewered meat dish known as Shish Kebab (page 143), also has the makings of a classic.

The Marinade:
⅔ cup olive oil
Juice of 5 - 6 lemons
1 teaspoon dry mustard
¼ teaspoon ground cumin
¼ teaspoon salt
½ teaspoon ground black pepper

The Fish:
1 pound swordfish steaks, cut into 1-inch cubes
1 small eggplant, peeled and cut into 1-inch cubes
Salt
1 - 2 tablespoons olive oil
3 tablespoons sesame seeds
1 lemon, cut in wedges

Special Equipment:
6 wooden skewers, soaked in cold water for 1 hour, or metal skewers

1. Combine all of the marinade ingredients in a non-metallic bowl. Toss in fish cubes. Cover and refrigerate for at least 1 hour before cooking.
2. Soak the eggplant cubes in heavily salted cold water for at least 15 minutes. This removes any bitterness from the eggplant and helps firm the fruit for grilling. Drain and pat dry with paper towels.
3. Set two shallow dishes next to each other in your work area. Pour the olive oil in one dish and the sesame seeds in the other. Roll each cube of

eggplant in olive oil, then coat with seeds. Skewer the sesame-seed–covered eggplant cubes on sticks.

4. Remove the fish cubes from the marinade and thread them evenly on skewers also.

5. Prepare the grill for cooking and lightly oil the grill rack. Grill the fish and eggplant skewers next to each other over a medium-hot fire. Turn each skewer, cooking evenly, until just cooked through. The fish will take about 6 minutes total; the eggplant may take slightly longer.

Note: This recipe also works well with tuna or mako shark. If you are not able to grill, brochettes can be broiled on an oiled broiler rack set about 4 inches from the heat, turning once, until just cooked through. Cooking times should be about the same as if grilling.

✑ Sesame Salmon Fillets with Tahini Sauce ✑

Serves 2

Pretty, pink, succulent salmon fries up firm and juicy when coated with the toasty crunch of sesame seeds. Served on a bed of rich, earthy tahini sauce, this dish is gourmet all the way. For dessert, offer Tahini Paklava (page 240), especially if serving this dish during Lent.

The Sauce:
¾ cup Tahini Sauce (page 225)

The Fish:
1 pound fresh salmon fillet, cut into individual serving size fillets, skin removed
¼ cup water (use milk if it's not Lent)
6 tablespoons white all-purpose flour
¼ teaspoon salt
¼ cup sesame seeds
2 tablespoons vegetable oil
1 lemon, cut in wedges
Fresh flat-leaf parsley

Special Equipment:
Meat mallet

1. Prepare the tahini sauce as per instructions.
2. Rinse the fish under cold running water; pat dry with paper towels. If the fillets are thicker than ½-inch, place one fillet at a time between pieces of clear plastic wrap. Gently pound the fish with the flat side of a meat mallet, working from the center out to the edges, until the fillet is an even thickness, about ½-inch. If necessary, trim to tidy the fillet edges before setting them aside.
3. Place water (or milk) in a shallow dish.
4. Combine the flour, salt, and sesame seeds in a second shallow dish.
5. Heat the oil in a large skillet until it's hot but not smoking.

6. Dip the salmon fillets in the liquid, then firmly press each side of the fillet into the sesame seed mixture.

7. Place the coated fillets in the skillet and cook 4 to 6 minutes on one side, then turn them over, and cook until the fish just begins to flake, about 2 more minutes.

8. Drizzle a spoonful of tahini sauce on an individual dinner plate and place a fillet on top. Garnish with lemon wedges and parsley. These fillets are delicious served with pilaf and a simple tossed green salad.

ARMENIAN
BASICS

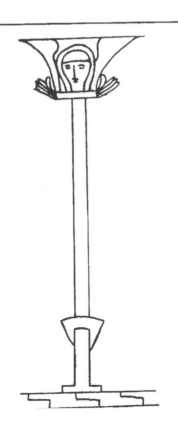

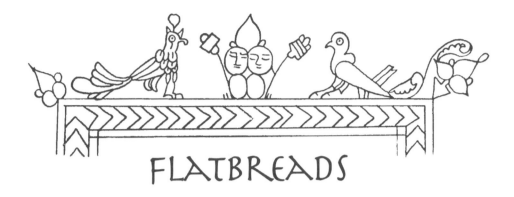

FLATBREADS

Armenian Cracker Bread

Makes 8 rounds

Armenian cracker bread is the most basic bread in the Armenian kitchen and the bread that supposedly almost did in my great-great-grandmother (see page 227).

Growing up, we called it "Bubble Bread," because these thin, round, brittle loaves sprinkled with sesame seeds are polka-dotted with golden-brown bubbles that are fun to crack with your thumb.

For years we bought loaves at the Middle Eastern store, and if the store was out we went without. But since I figured out how easy it is to make, my family has never been without "Bubble Bread." My daughter and I often bake this bread as a rainy-day-afternoon project because it's as much fun to make as it is to eat.

The Dough:
1⅓ cups warm water (about 105 degrees)
¼ cup olive oil, plus additional to grease bowl
3 tablespoons sugar
1 package (¼ ounce) active dry yeast
2 teaspoons salt
4 cups white bread flour, plus additional for rolling

The Topping:
½ cup whole milk
Sesame seeds

Special Equipment:
Tabletop mixer with batter blade and dough hook
(optional but recommended)
Heavy rolling pin

1. Put the water, olive oil, sugar, and yeast in the bowl of a tabletop electric mixer. Using the batter blade, let the mixer blend these well, about 5 minutes on low speed. Stir in the salt. (If making by hand, blend with a wooden spoon.)

2. Gradually add 2 cups of flour and beat on low speed until a thick, smooth dough forms. Change the blade to a dough hook and knead in the next 2 cups of flour. Continue kneading with the dough hook for 10 minutes. (By hand, mix the dough in a large mixing bowl and then knead it on a floured work surface for 20 minutes until smooth and elastic.)

3. Place the dough in a large bowl generously coated with olive oil, turning once to cover with oil. Cover loosely with a clean kitchen cloth and set in a warm place until the dough doubles in bulk, about 1½ hours.

4. Turn the dough out onto a floured work surface and punch down. Divide into 8 equal pieces. Cover and let stand for 15 minutes.

5. Preheat the oven to 375 degrees.

6. On a well-floured work surface, roll out each piece of dough into a 12-inch-diameter circle. Arrange the rounds on ungreased baking sheets. Brush with milk, sprinkle sesame seeds over the top, and brush again to secure the seeds.

7. With a fork, prick each round many times, all over. Pricking makes the bubbles appear. If you forget this step the loaf will puff up like a balloon.

8. Bake in the middle of the oven for 8 to 10 minutes, or until lightly browned on top.

9. This Armenian dietary cornerstone can be eaten as a cracker topped with honey, peanut butter, jelly, tomatoes, or cucumbers. Or, when moistened with water, it becomes soft and pliable enough to roll up sandwich goodies inside like a wrap.

Toasted Pita Chips

Serves 8

Americans have wholeheartedly embraced pita bread. Fresh loaves can be found in supermarkets across the country, so it's not necessary to make it from scratch. But go the extra distance and make your own pita chips—because they're easy and they're scrumptious.

4 large pita bread rounds
Olive oil
Finely shredded parmesan cheese (optional)

1. Preheat the oven to 350 degrees.
2. Split the pita loaf into two rounds. Sometimes this process is easier if the bread is heated in the microwave on high for 10 seconds first.
3. Brush the insides of each round with olive oil. Sprinkle cheese evenly over the round (if desired) and place it, cut side up, in a single layer on a baking sheet. (If the rounds overlap, be sure to separate them immediately after baking or they will stick together as they cool.)
4. Bake in the middle of the oven for 10 minutes or until golden. Allow the rounds to cool before breaking into chips.
5. These toasted chips may be served immediately with your favorite spread or stored at room temperature in an airtight container; pita chips will stay fresh for up to a week.

Butter-Flake Bread

This bread is the perfect breakfast treat, especially when served with cheese or preserves.

The Dough:
1 package (¼ ounce) active dry yeast
¼ cup warm water (about 105 degrees)
4 cups white bread flour, plus additional for rolling
1 cup warm evaporated milk (about 105 degrees)
1 large egg, beaten
1 teaspoon salt
1 tablespoon sugar
4 tablespoons (½ stick) unsalted butter, melted, plus 1 tablespoon
unsalted butter, melted, for greasing bowl, and ¼ pound (1 stick)
unsalted butter, melted

The Topping:
1 large egg, beaten
Sesame seeds

Special Equipment:
Tabletop mixer with dough hook (optional)
Heavy rolling pin

1. Stir the yeast into the water in a small, non-metallic mixing bowl until it dissolves. Set aside.
2. Sift the flour into a large mixing bowl. Remove 1 cup and set aside. Gently make a hole in the center of the remaining flour.
3. Combine the evaporated milk, egg, salt, and sugar in a third bowl. Whisk until well blended. Pour the milk mixture into the center of the flour. Add the yeast. Gently combine until the mixture is the consistency of a thin paste. Cover and leave in a warm place for 10 minutes or until the yeast froths.

4. Beat the dough, vigorously, by hand for 2 minutes. Gradually add the 4 tablespoons melted butter along with the 1 cup of flour that was set aside in step 2.

5. Turn the dough into the bowl of an electric mixer and beat with a dough hook for 5 minutes or knead by hand for the same amount of time.

6. Turn the dough out onto a lightly floured work surface. Continue to work the dough for 10 minutes until it is satiny smooth; add more flour if necessary. Then form into a ball. Grease a large bowl generously with 1 tablespoon melted butter. Place the dough in the bowl, turning once to coat it with butter. Cover, and let the dough rise in a warm place for 1 hour or until doubled in size.

7. Punch dough down and turn it onto a lightly floured work surface. Divide into 6 equal portions. Cover loosely with a clean kitchen towel.

8. Taking 1 piece at a time, roll the dough into large, wafer-thin circles, about 16 inches in diameter. Brush the circles evenly with the remaining ¼ pound melted butter. Roll each circle into a long rope shape. Holding each end, beat each rope on the work surface until it stretches to twice its original length.

9. Coil the dough ropes into rounds, tucking the ends into the centers. (The rounds will look like cinnamon rolls.) Flatten slightly with your hands.

10. When all the dough is shaped, use a rolling pin to flatten each coil into a 7-inch round. Place each round on a greased baking sheet. Cover loosely with a clean kitchen towel and leave to rise for 45 minutes or until doubled in size.

11. Preheat the oven to 375 degrees.

12. Brush the doubled rounds with egg, sprinkle with sesame seeds, and brush with egg again to secure the seeds. Bake each round in the middle of the oven for 12 to 15 minutes, until golden on top.

13. Cool to room temperature before serving with more butter (if you dare!) or a slice of cheese or spoonful of your favorite preserve.

Butter-Layered Flatbread

Pagharch

Makes 6 loaves

My husband's Auntie Payloun shared her family-famous recipe for pagharch bread with me. Although similar to the Butter-Flake Bread (page 192), the texture of these loaves is more layered than flaky. Thanks, Auntie!

The Dough:
5 pounds white bread flour (about 16⅔ cups)
1 package (¼ ounce) active dry yeast
2 teaspoons baking powder
1 teaspoon salt
1 cup whole milk
1 cup water
¼ pound (1 stick) butter
½ cup solid shortening
5 large eggs
½ pound (2 sticks) butter, melted

The Topping:
1 large egg
1 tablespoon whole milk
Sesame seeds

Special Equipment:
Tabletop mixer with dough hook (optional)
Heavy rolling pin

1. Combine 6 cups of the flour with the yeast, baking powder, and salt in a large mixing bowl. Set aside.
2. Heat the milk, water, ¼ pound butter, and solid shortening in a saucepan over low heat, stirring frequently, until the fats are just melted, about 105 degrees.

3. Pour the warmed liquid into the flour and mix to a paste. Add the eggs. Gradually add the additional 4 cups of flour, mixing well between each addition. Transfer the dough to the bowl of a tabletop mixer. Using the dough hook, mix for 5 minutes or knead the dough by hand on a lightly floured work surface until it is soft, smooth, and elastic, about 10 minutes.

4. Divide into 6 balls. Cover with a clean kitchen towel and put in a warm place for about 1½ hours, or until the balls double in size.

5. Roll each ball separately on a spacious, well-floured work surface until the dough is as thin as possible. In the old days, Armenian women used a long wooden dowel to roll the dough paper-thin. A heavy rolling pin works just as well.

6. Once rolled, brush the entire surface with melted butter (½ pound). Fold each side of the dough into the center. Butter again. Fold and butter, until the final fold makes a loaf measuring about 8-inches square. Lightly roll out the loaf square into an 8 x 12-inch rectangle. Set aside on a baking sheet.

7. Preheat the oven to 350 degrees. Repeat steps 5 and 6 until all loaves are buttered and folded.

8. Combine the egg and milk in a small dish. Brush the top of each loaf with egg wash, sprinkle sesame seeds on top, and brush again with egg to secure the seeds. Set in a warm place and allow each loaf to rise again, covered, for 20 minutes.

9. Bake in the middle of the oven until both the top and bottom are browned, about 35 minutes.

10. Serve with Armenian string cheese for breakfast or as a midmorning or midafternoon snack with coffee.

Note: Loaves freeze well in airtight plastic freezer bags.

Flapjack Skillet Bread

Saji Hatz

Makes 24 loaves

Rolling out dough is fast becoming a lost art. Sippy Andonian of the Whitinsville, Massachusetts, Armenian Church Ladies Guild is a master. She tells stories about how her mother stood over her shoulder, instructing and watching and correcting her as a young girl, until she could roll dough 5 feet in diameter across the table with a dowel. In those days (not that long ago!) paper-thin pastry layers were a matter of pride.

When Sippy and her gang of church ladies make this flatbread for their annual bazaar, they make 125 loaves! Even cut to 2 dozen, this recipe is a lot of work and best done with at least one kitchen partner. (The recipe yields enough to share.)

Similar in taste to some of the other buttery flatbreads found in this collection, these loaves are not baked but cooked on a griddle, which gives them an edgy hot-off-the-grill flavor that is distinctive and really outstanding.

I am grateful to Sippy for sharing this recipe with me, and with you.

The Dough:
5 pounds white bread flour (about 16⅔ cups)
3 tablespoons butter, softened
3 tablespoons solid shortening
1 package (¼ ounce) active dry yeast
1 tablespoon sugar
1 teaspoon salt
3 cups warm water (about 105 degrees)

The Filling:
1 tablespoon butter, melted for greasing bowl, plus 1 pound (4 sticks) butter, melted

Special Equipment:
Tabletop mixer with dough hook (optional)
Heavy rolling pin
Gas oven or flapjack griddle

1. Combine the flour, 3 tablespoons softened butter, shortening, yeast, sugar, and salt in a jumbo-sized mixing bowl. Cut the fats into the flour with a large fork until evenly distributed.
2. Slowly stir the warm water into the flour.
3. Turn the dough out onto a well-floured work surface and knead by hand until the dough is soft and smooth. If using a tabletop mixer, depending on its capacity, the dough may need to be divided into parts. Mix each part in the mixer with the dough hook for 5 minutes, then knead the balls into one large ball by hand on a floured work surface until soft and smooth. Place the dough in a well-buttered bowl, cover loosely with a clean kitchen towel, and place the bowl in a warm place until it doubles in size, about 1½ hours. If necessary, separate the dough into two halves during this step also.
4. Turn the dough out onto a floured work surface and punch it down. Divide the dough into 24 (3-inch) balls. Knead each ball until smooth. Set the balls aside in a warm place covered with a towel to rise again.
5. On a large floured work surface, roll out 1 ball at a time as thin as possible into an oval. Don't worry if a few holes open up. It's even fine to pull the dough gently with the palms of your hands. The important thing is to roll the pastry as thin as possible—thin enough to have made Sippy's mother proud!
6. Once the dough is rolled, brush the oval with melted butter. Fold the bottom edge up to the middle and the top edge down to meet it. Butter again. Fold the left edge into the center and the right edge in to meet it. Butter again. Continue to fold and butter until each sheet becomes a 4-inch square. Then, twist the square into a ball. Set the ball on a baking sheet, then repeat until all the dough has been rolled, buttered, and reshaped into buttery balls.
7. If using a gas stove, preheat the oven to 475 - 500 degrees. If using a flapjack griddle, preheat it to the same temperature.

8. Roll each buttery ball out again on your work surface into an 8 x 12-inch rectangular loaf.

9. Place each loaf directly on the bottom of the oven or on top of the hot griddle. Grill until brown on one side, about 2 minutes. Then flip the loaf over and cook until brown on the other side. Cool on a wire rack.

10. Serve cooled with cheese or tear off a piece and just eat it plain. Yum! This flatbread is my personal favorite.

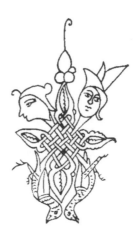

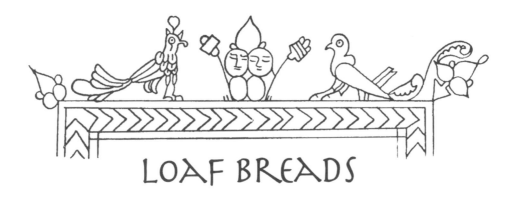

LOAF BREADS

Cracked Wheat Bread

Makes 2 loaves

1 cup coarse-grain bulgur
3¾ to 4½ cups white bread flour, plus additional for kneading
1 package (¼ ounce) active dry yeast
¼ cup sugar
1 tablespoon butter
1 teaspoon salt
1¼ cups whole wheat bread flour
¼ cup unprocessed wheat bran (see Note)
Olive oil

Special Equipment:
Tabletop mixer with dough hook (optional)
2 (8 x 4-inch) loaf pans

1. Stir 2 cups of boiling water into the bulgur in a medium-sized mixing bowl. Let stand for 5 minutes. Drain off excess water and set aside.
2. Combine 1½ cups of the white flour and yeast in a second large mixing bowl. Set aside. (If you are using a tabletop mixer, put the flour in the mixer's bowl and use the dough hook in steps 4 and 5.)
3. Heat 1¾ cups water in a saucepan until just warm. Add the sugar, butter, and salt. Stir until the butter is almost melted. Take care not to overheat

the mixture. Too much heat will kill the active yeast. Just warm and comfortable to the touch, like a newborn baby's first bath, about 105 degrees.

4. Pour the warmed butter mixture into the flour. Beat on low for 30 seconds, then on high for 3 minutes. Scrape the sides of the bowl as often as necessary. Then use a wooden spoon to stir in the drained bulgur, whole-wheat flour, and wheat bran. Finally, add the remaining white flour.

5. Turn the dough out onto a floured work surface. Knead for about 6 to 8 minutes by hand or 5 minutes in the bowl of a tabletop mixer with a dough hook. Add additional flour, as needed, to make a smooth and elastic yet moderately stiff dough. Shape the dough into a ball and place in a bowl lightly greased with olive oil. Turn once to coat completely. Cover with a clean kitchen towel and set to rise in a warm place till doubled in size, about 1¼ hours.

6. Turn the dough out onto a floured work surface and punch down. Divide in half and reshape into two balls of equal size. Cover again loosely with a towel and let rest for 10 minutes.

7. Lightly grease the two loaf pans with olive oil. Reshape each ball of dough to fit into the prepared pans. Cover with a towel, and set in a warm place, letting the dough rise again until nearly doubled in size, about 40 minutes.

8. Preheat the oven to 375 degrees.

9. Bake the loaves in the middle of the oven for 35 to 40 minutes, or until the bread sounds hollow when tapped on top with the back of a spoon. Remove the loaves from the pans immediately and cool completely on a wire rack.

10. Serve sliced with cheese or to complement a hearty soup or salad.

Note: Unprocessed wheat bran can be found in health food or whole food grocery stores, usually sold in bulk bins.

Savory Dill Bread

Makes 1 loaf

The Dough:
1 package (¼ ounce) active dry yeast
¼ cup warm water (about 105 degrees)
2 tablespoons sugar
1 cup small-curd cottage cheese
1 tablespoon minced dried onion
1 tablespoon butter
2 teaspoons dried dill seeds
1 teaspoon salt
¼ teaspoon baking soda
1 large egg, slightly beaten
2¼ to 2½ cups white bread flour, plus additional for kneading
Olive oil

The Topping:
1 teaspoon butter, melted
½ teaspoon dried dill seeds

Special Equipment:
1 (9 x 5-inch) loaf pan, greased with olive oil

1. Combine the yeast, warm water, and 1 tablespoon of the sugar in a small, non-metallic bowl. Whisk well before setting the mixture aside until the yeast froths, about 10 minutes.
2. Meanwhile, in a saucepan combine the cottage cheese, the remaining tablespoon sugar, onion, butter, dill seeds, salt, and baking soda. Heat, stirring continuously, until the butter is just melted, about 105 degrees. Remove from heat.
3. Combine the yeast with the cheese mixture in a large mixing bowl. Add the egg. Then stir in as much of the flour as possible.
4. Turn the dough out onto a floured work surface. Knead in the remaining flour, making a moderately soft, smooth, elastic dough. A total of 3 to 5

minutes of kneading should be enough. Shape the dough into a ball. Place it in a large bowl generously coated with olive oil, turning the dough once to coat with oil on all sides.

5. Cover with a clean kitchen towel and let the dough rise in a warm place until doubled in size, about 1½ hours.

6. Turn the dough out onto a floured work surface and punch it down. Shape the dough and place it into the prepared pan. Cover and let it rise again in a warm place until nearly doubled in size, about 40 minutes.

7. Preheat the oven to 350 degrees.

8. Brush the top of the loaf with the melted butter, sprinkle with dill seed, and brush with butter again to secure the seeds.

9. Bake in the middle of the oven for 40 to 45 minutes or until the loaf is golden brown and the bread sounds hollow when tapped on the top with the back of a spoon. If necessary, cover the bread loosely with foil for the last 15 minutes of baking to prevent over-browning.

10. Immediately remove the bread from the pan and cool completely on a wire rack before serving.

11. This bread is a perfect complement to the soups and stews of the Armenian kitchen.

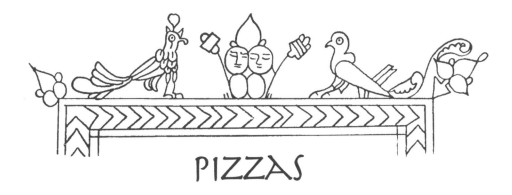

PIZZAS

Armenian Meat Pizza

Lahmejun

Makes 12

It's possible that these pizzas, known in Armenian as lahmejun (from the Arabic "lahm wa ajeen," meaning meat and bread), look and taste like the first pizzas in the history of world cuisine. Reportedly originating in Babylon, thin-crust pizzas were eaten by sheiks as they crossed the desert. When the caravan stopped for the night, the women would prepare the dough from starter they carried with them. One of the lambs that marched along with the caravan would be butchered, and the meat ground. Then a sheet of metal was placed over the campfire and these pizzas would be prepared fresh and served as the evening meal.

While they may have been made and served for centuries, given that these pizzas freeze well and heat up quickly (warmed at 350 degrees for four minutes)—they also seem very contemporary, even hip. They are floppy and fun to roll up like a wrap, and their slightly spicy flavor hits the spot for a light lunch, an after-school snack, or when cut in wedges and served as an appetizer.

You can buy these pizzas ready-made in Armenian markets from Los Angeles to New York, or for some real fun try making your own. My recipe is worth the effort.

The Dough:
1 package (¼ ounce) active dry yeast
1 cup warm water (about 105 degrees)
1 tablespoon olive oil, plus additional for greasing bowl and
baking sheets
½ teaspoon sugar
¼ teaspoon salt
2¼ cups white bread flour, plus additional for rolling

The Topping:
1 pound ground lamb
1 can (14½ ounces) tomatoes, peeled, diced, and drained well
2 tablespoons tomato paste
½ red pepper, finely chopped
½ green pepper, finely chopped
½ onion, finely chopped
⅓ cup finely chopped fresh flat-leaf parsley
1 teaspoon salt
½ teaspoon ground black pepper
¼ teaspoon crushed red pepper flakes
¼ teaspoon cayenne
Fresh lemon juice

Special Equipment:
Tabletop mixer with dough hook (optional)
Food processor or blender
Heavy rolling pin

1. To prepare the dough, dissolve the yeast in water in the bowl of the tabletop mixer. Stir in the 1 tablespoon olive oil, sugar, salt, and 1½ cups flour. Mix the dough with a dough hook until smooth, about 3 minutes. Knead in the remaining flour until the dough is smooth and elastic. This will take about 10 minutes by machine, 20 minutes by hand.
2. Shape the dough into a ball and place in a large bowl greased with olive oil. Turn the ball once to coat it completely with oil. Cover with a clean

kitchen towel and let stand in a warm place for about 1½ hours, or until doubled in size.

3. While waiting for the dough to rise, combine all of the topping ingredients together in the bowl of a food processor (or blender) and pulse until just smooth. Set aside.

4. When the dough has doubled in size, turn it out onto a floured work surface and punch it down. Knead the dough into the shape of a log. Cut the log into 12 equal pieces. Then roll each piece out into a 7-inch circle.

5. Preheat the oven to 375 degrees.

6. Lightly grease 2 to 4 baking sheets with olive oil. Arrange the circles on the prepared baking sheets. Allow the dough to rest and rise slightly, about 15 minutes. Then, spread the meat mixture evenly over the entire surface of each round.

7. Bake in the middle of the oven for 25 to 30 minutes. Cool the pizzas on a wire rack.

8. Serve warm with a splash of fresh lemon juice for a quick lunch or snack.

Green Onion and Pine Nut Pizza

Makes 8 pizzas

These vegetarian pizzas are soft yet crispy, and their golden-brown bubbles covered with green and white scallions and pine nuts are as beautiful to look at as they are yummy. The taste is so authentic that taking your first bite is like a trip to the old country.

The Dough:
1 package (¼ ounce) active dry yeast
1 teaspoon sugar
¼ cup whole milk, at room temperature
2½ cups white bread flour, plus additional for rolling
½ cup warm water (about 105 degrees)
2 tablespoons unsalted butter, melted
½ teaspoon salt
Olive oil

The Topping:
4 tablespoons (½ stick) unsalted butter
½ cup raw pine nuts, coarsely chopped
16 scallions (white and light green part only), thinly sliced (about 2 cups)
¼ cup finely chopped fresh flat-leaf parsley
½ teaspoon salt
¼ teaspoon ground black pepper

Special Equipment:
Heavy rolling pin

1. Begin making the dough by whisking the yeast, sugar, and milk together in a small non-metallic bowl until the yeast dissolves. Set aside until the mixture froths, about 10 minutes.
2. Transfer the frothy mixture to a large mixing bowl and add the flour, water, butter, and salt. Mix to form a ball. Turn the ball out onto a floured work surface and knead until smooth and supple, about 5 minutes.

3. Place in a bowl oiled with olive oil; turn to coat. Cover with a clean kitchen towel and let rise in a warm place for about 1½ hours.

4. While the dough is rising, prepare the topping. Melt the butter in a saucepan over medium heat. Add the pine nuts; cook, stirring, until the nuts are lightly golden, 1 to 2 minutes. Add the scallions and parsley. Cook until the scallions are soft, about 4 minutes, and then season with salt and pepper.

5. Preheat the oven to 500 degrees.

6. Turn the doubled-in-size dough out onto a floured work surface. Punch down and reshape into a log. Divide the dough log into 8 pieces. Roll and flatten each piece on a floured work surface into a 7-inch long and 4-inch wide, elliptical shape. Spread the onion mixture generously down the center of each piece.

7. Place pizzas on a baking sheet, 2 at a time. Bake in the middle of the oven until lightly golden, 5 to 7 minutes.

8. For a crispy pizza, serve immediately. For a softer variety, stack the pizzas on a wire rack, cover with a clean kitchen towel, and let rest for 5 minutes. Fantastic when served with a medley of salads.

✥ Zahtar Bread ✥

Makes 8

Zahtar is a thyme-like herb that is often blended with sumac bark and chickpeas or sesame seeds. It is imported from Lebanon, Syria, and Jordan and sold in Middle Eastern markets. Often, those markets also sell packages of freshly prepared zahtar bread. You can explore its unique taste by trying a bakery-made loaf, but making it at home is better because the packaged breads are sometimes heavy, both on taste and the tummy.

The Dough:
6 cups white bread flour, plus additional for rolling
1 package (¼ ounce) active dry yeast
2 cups warm water (about 105 degrees)
1½ teaspoons salt
1 teaspoon sugar
2 tablespoons olive oil, plus additional for greasing

The Topping:
1 cup zahtar
1⅓ cups extra-virgin olive oil

Special Equipment:
Tabletop mixer with dough hook (optional)
Heavy rolling pin

1. Sift the flour into a large mixing bowl and warm in a low oven.
2. Dissolve the yeast in ¼ cup of the warmed water in a non-metallic bowl. Once the yeast is dissolved, add the remaining water and stir in the salt and sugar.
3. Place about 2 cups of the warmed flour in the mixing bowl of a tabletop mixer or in a large mixing bowl if you are preparing the dough by hand. Pour the yeast liquid into the center of the flour and stir with a wooden spoon to make a thick paste. Cover with a clean kitchen towel and put in a warm place until the mixture froths, about 10 minutes.

4. Stir in 3 additional cups of flour. Add the olive oil gradually, mixing after each addition. Knead the dough until smooth, either by hand for 10 minutes or in the mixer with a dough hook for 5 minutes.

5. Turn the dough out onto a floured work surface and knead for 10 minutes; use the reserved flour as required. The dough is ready when it is smooth and satiny and has a slightly wrinkled texture. Shape into a ball.

6. Place the dough in a large bowl greased with olive oil; turn it once to coat. Cover with a clean kitchen towel and leave in a warm place to rise until almost doubled in size, about 1 to 1½ hours.

7. Turn the dough out onto a floured work surface and punch down. Knead for a minute or so, then divide into 8 equal pieces. Shape each piece into a ball.

8. Roll each ball flat into a 10-inch round disk. Place each round on a lightly floured clean kitchen towel. Cover with another towel and leave for 20 minutes to rise.

9. Preheat the oven to 500 degrees. Place baking sheets inside the oven to preheat them.

10. Make the topping in a small bowl by mixing the olive oil and zahtar together. Taking 1 round at a time, flute the edges, then brush a generous spoonful of zahtar evenly over the top.

11. Rub the heated baking sheet with a wad of paper towel dipped in olive oil. Place a round of dough onto the prepared baking sheet. Bake in the middle of the hot oven for 5 minutes, or until the bread puffs up like a balloon.

12. Cool on a wire rack while baking the remaining loaves similarly.

13. Eat immediately or store the cooled breads in an airtight container. Zahtar bread is best served at room temperature as a between-meal snack or alongside a tossed green salad for lunch.

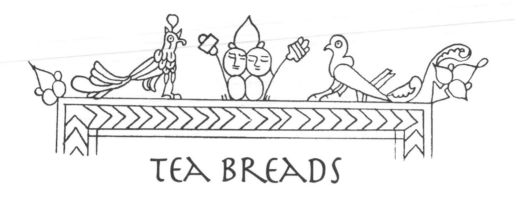

TEA BREADS

Tea Rolls

Choreg

Makes 24

For centuries, Armenian women have combined milk, butter, eggs, and a bit of sugar with yeast dough to bake sweet rolls called choregs. Who makes the best choreg is a never-ending topic of debate in every Armenian family. In my family, some say it was my grandmother; others insist my aunt wins first prize.

As with all bread-making, ferreting out the secrets of good choreg baking is no easy task. Factor in humidity, temperature, and all the other variables that plague artisan bread makers, and even a great recipe can disappoint. My recipe is an amalgamation of family secrets and experimentation designed to allow for worry-free preparation and rave reviews.

I use two ingredients not commonly found in the American spice pantry to obtain the unique flavor of my choregs—mahleb and nigella seeds. Mahleb is ground black cherry pits and nigella seeds are strong-flavored black caraway seeds. Both are available in Middle Eastern markets.

The Dough:
½ package (⅛ ounce) active dry yeast
¼ cup warm water (about 105 degrees)
5 - 6 cups white bread flour
⅓ cup sugar

1 teaspoon ground mahleb
½ teaspoon salt
2 cups whole milk
⅜ pound (1½ sticks) butter
2 large eggs, beaten
½ teaspoon nigella seeds (optional)
Olive oil

The Topping:
1 large egg, beaten
Sesame seeds

Special Equipment:
Tabletop mixer with dough hook (optional)

1. Dissolve the yeast in the water in a small non-metallic bowl. Set aside.
2. Combine 5 cups of flour, sugar, ground mahleb, and salt in a large mixing bowl or in the bowl of a tabletop mixer.
3. Place the milk and butter in a saucepan and heat until the butter just melts, about 105 degrees. Pour the warmed liquid into the flour mixture. Mix well before adding the eggs, and the nigella seeds, if desired.
4. Knead the dough 5 minutes in the mixer with a dough hook or 10 minutes by hand on a floured work surface. The dough will be sticky; wetting your hands with warm water will help you work with it. If the dough is too sticky, add additional flour. Depending on the day's humidity, an additional 1 to 1½ cups of flour may be needed to make sure the dough is stiff enough to retain its shape in a ball.
5. Shape the dough into a large ball. Place it in a jumbo-sized bowl greased with olive oil; turn to coat. Cover the bowl with a clean kitchen towel and place it in a warm place. Let rise for 1½ hours, until dough doubles in size.
6. Turn the dough out onto a floured work surface, punch down, and reshape it into a ball. Divide the dough in half with a sharp knife. Then divide each half into 12 pieces. Roll each of the 24 pieces out into rope, about ½-inch thick. Wind each rope cinnamon roll-style into a bun.
7. Place the buns on large baking sheets; 12 to a sheet. Cover each sheet with a clean kitchen towel. Put in a warm place and let rise for 20 minutes.

8. Preheat the oven to 375 degrees.
9. Brush the top of each roll with egg. Sprinkle with sesame seeds and brush the top again to secure the seeds.
10. Bake in the middle of the oven for about 20 minutes or until the rolls are golden brown.
11. Delicious served with cheese or your favorite preserves.

Variation: **Chocolate Chip Choreg**

If the French can stuff croissants with chocolate, then the Armenians can put chocolate chips in their choregs. Knead 1 cup mini chocolate chips into the dough after the first rising and before coiling into individual rolls. Truly outstanding!

Armenian–Jam–Filled Muffins

Makes 12

Breakfasts are made special when serving muffins stuffed with Armenian-made apricot or peach jam. What a great way to support Armenia—by using a delicious product made and exported from the country. So delight your family with these lemon-flavored breakfast cakes filled with a sweet, and maybe a little sticky, surprise inside. They'll love it!

1¾ cups white all-purpose flour
½ cup sugar
1 tablespoon baking powder
½ teaspoon salt
2 large eggs
⅓ cup butter, melted
1 teaspoon grated lemon peel
½ cup Armenian-made apricot or peach jam

Special Equipment:
12-muffin pan, grease or paper-line the cups

1. Preheat the oven to 400 degrees.
2. Combine the flour, sugar, baking powder, and salt in a large mixing bowl.
3. In a smaller bowl, lightly beat the eggs. Stir in the melted butter and lemon peel. Add to the flour and blend just until moistened.
4. Spoon half of the batter into the prepared muffin cups. Moistening your fingers with warm water may help you spread the batter evenly in the cup and make a well in the center of each. (Be sure to use only half the batter for the bottom layer. The layer may seem shallow, but that's okay. You need the other half for the top, so be conservative.)
5. Spoon a dollop of jam into each muffin well. Cover the jam with the remaining batter.
6. Bake in the middle of the oven for 20 minutes or until golden on top.
7. Serve along with coffee or as a complement to eggs.

Sesame Cookies

Simit

Makes 4 dozen

These cookies are easy to prepare and great to have on hand. Not too sweet, but not savory either, they go nicely with coffee, tea, or ice-cold milk. They are the perfect "little something" to have on hand to serve drop-in guests.

3 cups sifted white all-purpose flour
3 teaspoons baking powder
2 tablespoons sugar
1½ teaspoons salt
¾ cup solid shortening
3 tablespoons dark corn syrup
½ cup cold milk
1 large egg, beaten
¾ cup sesame seeds

1. Preheat the oven to 300 degrees.
2. Combine the flour, baking powder, sugar, and salt in a large mixing bowl.
3. Using a large fork, cut the shortening into the flour until the mixture has the texture of meal. Add the corn syrup and mix well. Then sprinkle the milk into the dough; mix thoroughly. If necessary, add a little more milk to make the dough medium-stiff yet easy to roll.
4. Take a small ball of dough and warm it in the palm of your hands, then roll it out on a flat work surface into a long pencil-thick strip. Fold the dough in half and twist like a hairpin, about 3-inches long. Arrange the cookies on ungreased baking sheets.
5. Brush each cookie with egg. Sprinkle with sesame seeds, then brush again with egg to secure the seeds. Bake in the middle of the oven for 25 to 30 minutes or until golden on top. Remove the cookies immediately from the cookie sheets to a wire rack to cool. The cookies have a tendency to stick if left to cool on the tray.
6. Stored in airtight containers; they will keep fresh for weeks.

Savory Cookies

Makes 5 dozen

My husband calls these savory snacks "Salty Cookies." This recipe requires mahleb and nigella seeds. Both ingredients are necessary to get the taste right. So head to the nearest Middle Eastern market or order them from one of the Mail-Order Sources (page 288).

6 cups white all-purpose flour
1 cup vegetable oil
1 cup warm water (about 105 degrees)
¼ pound (1 stick) butter, softened
½ cup solid shortening
1 tablespoon ground mahleb
1 tablespoon nigella seeds
1 tablespoon baking powder
1 tablespoon salt
1 large egg, beaten

1. Preheat the oven to 350 degrees.
2. Combine the flour, oil, water, butter, shortening, mahleb, nigella seeds, baking powder, and salt together in a large mixing bowl until smooth.
3. On a flat surface, roll a spoonful of dough at a time into a rope and join the ends to make a wreath-shaped cookie, measuring approximately 1½-inches in diameter.
4. Arrange the wreaths on an ungreased cookie sheet. Brush the top of each with beaten egg.
5. Bake in the middle of the oven for 25 minutes, or until golden brown.
6. Kept in an airtight container, these cookies will stay fresh for a long time.

Katah Sweet Rolls

Yields 4 to 6 dozen depending on size

I love this dough. It's soft and smooth and easy to work with, and best of all, you can prepare this recipe by hand.

The Dough:
2 packages (½ ounce) dry active yeast
2 cups sugar
¼ teaspoon ground ginger
8 heaping cups white bread flour, plus additional for rolling
1 pound (4 sticks) butter, melted
3 large eggs, plus 1 large egg, beaten for wash
2 cups warm whole milk (about 105 degrees)

Special Equipment:
Heavy rolling pin
3-inch-diameter round cookie cutter

1. Dissolve the yeast, 1 teaspoon sugar, and the ginger in ½ cup of warm water in a medium-sized non-metallic bowl. Set aside for at least 10 minutes to allow the yeast to froth.
2. In a large mixing bowl, combine the remaining sugar, flour, butter, 3 eggs, and milk until smooth. Add the yeast, kneading until the dough is smooth and the sides of the bowl are clean.
3. Turn the dough out onto a floured work surface. Knead in additional flour until the dough is firm enough to hold its shape as a large round. Cover with a clean kitchen towel and let the dough rise in a warm place for 3 hours.
4. Divide the dough into workable sections. Roll each section out to a ⅜-inch thickness on a floured work surface. Cut into individual circles with the cookie cutter. Set the rolls on a baking sheet, cover, and let rise again until double in size, about 1 hour.
5. Preheat the oven to 375 degrees.

6. Brush each roll with the remaining beaten egg and bake on ungreased baking sheets in the middle of the oven until golden brown on top, 12 to 15 minutes depending on size.

7. Serve these delicate sweet rolls for breakfast with cheese or jam, or for afternoon tea.

Note: I freeze the majority of this recipe's yield and defrost a few rolls at a time. That way I always have a quick breakfast treat or an accompaniment to an elaborate weekend brunch already prepared.

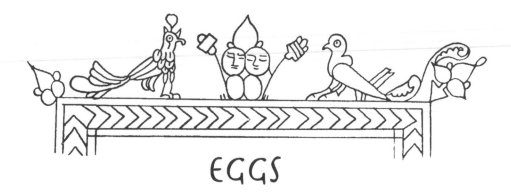

EGGS

Easter Eggs

1 dozen

It's Easter week. The Lenten fast is ending. Long before Christianity, the Hebrews, Assyrians, Egyptians, Persians, Greeks, Romans, Armenians, and other peoples prepared eggs on occasions of pomp and ceremony.

To them, the egg symbolized the Universe and was presented to their gods as an offering. The outer shell represented the limitless sky, and the inner skin the air. The white of the egg was the waters, and the yolk was the earth. Then, starting early in the Christian era, according to one legend, Mary Magdalene appeared in Rome before Emperor Tiberius. When she told him of the resurrection, he replied that a man could no more rise from the dead than turn an egg red. Mary picked up an egg and turned it red. Consequently, icons often depict her holding an egg, and Orthodox Christians color their Easter eggs red.

On Good Friday, my grandmother boiled her eggs in a huge blue-and-white speckled pot. Grandma liked her eggs dyed a deep garnet color, so after she turned off the heat, she left them to soak in the onion skins for a long time. I loved to poke my finger into the red juice and peek at the eggs hiding under the skins. To be fair, what I really wanted was to find the hardest-shelled egg and claim it as my own for the Easter Day Egg War. After our egg hunt, everyone in the family would take their strongest-looking egg and smash it against the crown of someone else's hardest egg. The egg that didn't crack won that battle, and the egg that did not crack in the whole family won the war.

As the only girl in a family of rough-and-tumble boy cousins, winning the Egg War was important to me.

Win or lose, it's traditions like egg dying, egg hunts, and egg wars that maintain the collective memory of any community. I offer this recipe as a reminder that continuing certain traditions is important. I also had to wear white gloves to church on Easter Sunday when I was a kid. Thankfully, some things do change!

12 large white-shelled eggs
Skins of yellow onions (see Step 1)
3 cups cold water
9 tablespoons white distilled vinegar
½ teaspoon salt

1. Start saving onion skins a few weeks ahead of time or buy a 5- to 10-pound bag of onions and slough off the outer layers of skins. (If you do, plan to use the onion soon because the skins help keep them fresh.)
2. Find a pot that will hold the eggs securely in one layer. Place the onion skins and the eggs in the pot.
3. In a separate bowl, combine the water, vinegar, and salt. Pour over eggs. The liquid should cover the eggs completely.
4. Bring quickly to a boil, lower the heat, and gently boil the eggs for about 10 minutes. Remove from heat. Let the eggs stand for at least 10 more minutes. At 10 minutes the eggs will be cooked to perfection for eating. If eating isn't your priority, well . . . let them sit a good long time for a rich brick-red color.

Scrambled Eggs with Apricots

Serves 2

Apricots (*Prunus armeniaca*) originated in Armenia. One August in Yerevan, I visited the Mardiros Saryan Museum and was offered a ripe apricot off the renowned painter's tree. It was juicy, sweet, and fragrant—like none other I have ever tasted. Fresh, or harvested and laid out to dry in the sun or strung to dry on strings like leis, Armenian apricots are heavenly.

1 tablespoon butter
¼ cup chopped onions
½ cup chopped dried apricots (about 6 dried fruits)
4 large eggs

1. Melt butter in a medium-sized skillet. Add the onions and sauté over moderate heat, stirring occasionally, until tender, about 10 minutes. Then add the apricots. Continue to cook, stirring occasionally, for another 5 minutes, until the apricots soften.
2. Meanwhile, beat the eggs thoroughly in a small mixing bowl. Pour the eggs into the skillet. Cook until light and fluffy, stirring frequently.
3. Serve this dish with Bulgur Pilaf (page 59) for a hearty breakfast, or as a light lunch or supper.

Spinach and Feta Cheese Omelet

Serves 2

This omelet starts any day off heartily. Consider it for a quick lunch or dinner, too.

10 ounces fresh spinach (about 8 cups), washed and trimmed of stems
1 tablespoon olive oil
¼ cup crumbled feta cheese
Pinch of salt
¼ teaspoon ground black pepper
Pinch of nutmeg (optional)
1 tablespoon butter
2 large eggs, beaten

1. Steam the spinach in a large deep-sided skillet with ¼ cup water over moderate heat until wilted, about 2 to 4 minutes. Rinse immediately in cold water and drain, pressing out excess liquid. Chop the spinach on a clean work surface.
2. Return the chopped spinach to the skillet, and add the olive oil, most of the cheese (put a pinch aside as topping), salt, black pepper, and nutmeg, if using. Sauté over medium-high heat for 3 minutes, stirring frequently.
3. Meanwhile, melt the butter over moderate heat in a smaller skillet, making sure the butter covers the bottom of the pan. Pour in the beaten eggs and cook until the eggs begin to firm, about 2 minutes. Then place the spinach mixture on top so that it covers the eggs evenly. Cover the pan, lower the heat, and cook until the egg layer is golden brown.
4. Flip at once onto a serving plate and serve egg side up, the top sprinkled with the reserved cheese and a turn of the pepper mill.

Scrambled Eggs with Soujouk

Serves 2

1 tablespoon butter
10 thin strips of Soujouk (page 39), cut into bite-sized pieces
4 large eggs
2 tablespoons milk

1. Melt the butter in a medium-sized skillet. Add the soujouk. Cook over moderate heat, stirring occasionally.
2. Beat the eggs and milk thoroughly in a small mixing bowl. Pour into the skillet. Cook eggs until light and fluffy, stirring constantly.
3. Serve hot with lots of pita bread.

Mashed Potatoes and Eggs

Serves 4

This is one of my husband's favorite dishes. This Armenian way to combine potatoes and eggs is delicious for breakfast, as a side, or even as a light meal.

3 medium-sized potatoes, peeled and cut into ¼-inch-thick slices (or start with leftover mashed potatoes)
Salt
3 tablespoons butter
2 tablespoons milk
2 large eggs
Sprinkle of cayenne

1. Place the potatoes in a large pot. Cover with water and salt to taste. Bring to a boil, lower the heat, and cook, slightly covered, until the potatoes are soft enough for a fork to easily break them apart, about 20 minutes. Remove from heat and drain.
2. Add 2 tablespoons butter and the milk. Mash with a potato masher, or better yet, whip the potatoes with an electric mixer. Set aside.
3. Whisk the eggs until frothy in a small mixing bowl. Then, in a medium-sized saucepan, melt the remaining 1 tablespoon butter over low heat, making sure the melted butter coats the bottom of the pan.
4. Pour the eggs into the pan and allow them to firm slightly, about 2 minutes, before spooning the mashed potatoes over the egg layer; gently pat the potatoes into an even layer. Cook another 2 minutes or so.
5. Flip onto a serving platter, egg side up. Garnish with cayenne. Slice in quarters and serve hot.

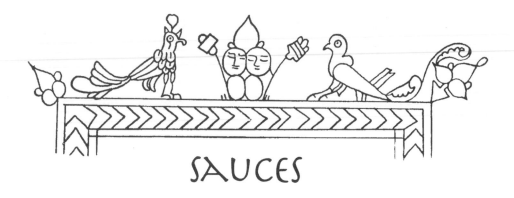

SAUCES

Balsamic Vinaigrette

Makes about ⅓ cup

This is my everyday household salad dressing. It's especially good with darker-leafed greens.

¼ cup extra-virgin olive oil
⅛ cup balsamic vinegar
½ teaspoon dry mustard
½ teaspoon salt
¼ teaspoon ground black pepper
1 whole garlic clove, cut in half

1. Whisk the oil, vinegar, mustard, salt, and pepper together in a small bowl. Add the garlic halves.
2. Remove the garlic after 30 minutes and before dressing the salad. Whisk again before using.

Note: Dressing can be made a day ahead of time.

Tahini Sauce

Makes ¾ cup

Tahini is a tan-colored paste made of toasted sesame seeds and sesame oil that has the consistency of natural peanut butter. It's found in Middle Eastern stores and in many supermarkets in the foreign foods section. This sauce complements most cooked or raw vegetables and fish.

1 small clove garlic
½ teaspoon salt
½ cup well-stirred tahini
Juice of 1 lemon
¼ cup cold water
Pinch of cayenne
3 pieces of roasted red pepper (optional)

Special Equipment:
Mortar and pestle
Blender (optional)

1. Grind the garlic clove with the salt in a mortar with a pestle.
2. Transfer the garlic paste to a small bowl. Stir in the tahini until well blended. Add a little water and a little lemon juice, alternately, until the sauce is the consistency desired. Once it is to your liking, add a pinch of cayenne to taste.
3. If using roasted red peppers, transfer the sauce to a blender, add the red peppers, and pulse until smooth. Adding red peppers gives the dressing a pretty pink hue but doesn't do much to the taste.
4. Serve at room temperature. Refrigerated, extra dressing keeps well for up to a week.

Yogurt Sauce

Makes 1 cup

1 cup plain yogurt
Juice of 1 lemon
¼ teaspoon salt
Pinch of cayenne
1 small garlic clove, pressed (optional)

1. In a small serving bowl, mix together the yogurt, lemon juice, salt, cayenne, and garlic, if using.
2. Served chilled or at room temperature. Delicious over grilled lamb.

Note: This dressing may be made a day ahead, covered, and chilled.

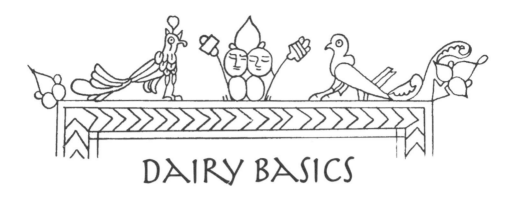

DAIRY BASICS

Homemade Yogurt

Madzoon

Makes 5 to 6 cups

Madzoon is the Armenian word for yogurt, which is derived from the Turkified Armenian word—yughort. Throughout the centuries, peoples from the Caucasus have consumed vast quantities of yogurt. They drink it (Tahn, page 231), eat it with cucumbers in a cool summer soup (Jajek, page 105), and often use it as a complement to other foods like meat-stuffed vegetables.

As a child, I was told that my great-great-grandmother once spent the day baking Armenian Cracker Bread (page 189) in her oven (tonir). She stacked the freshly baked rounds of bread in a basket as usual, but that night, a poisonous snake got into the basket and spit its venom on the rounds. The next day, when my great-great-grandmother ate the bread, she became very sick, poisoned by the snake. Her cure? A cup of yogurt. Soon thereafter, she made a full recovery.

I'm not sure if anyone really knows what saved my great-great-grandmother's life, but at the very least, the miracle properties of yogurt were indelibly impressed on me at a young age.

At one time in the United States, you could look in the phone book, locate a surname ending in -ian, call and ask the woman of the home for magart—yogurt starter—and you would find some! My grandmother and her generation of cooks were never without starter.

Homemade madzoon is delicious and simple to prepare. Be sure to clean your bowls and utensils well before starting. You want to cultivate the healthy bacteria in the yogurt, not random bacteria that may be present on the pots and utensils.

1 quart whole milk
1 - 2 tablespoons yogurt starter with active bacteria (see Note)

1. Pour the milk into a clean pot. Heat the milk to the scalding point—the point when it is ready to froth over the top of the pan. Immediately pour the scalded milk into a glass or ceramic container and let cool until temperate, about 105 degrees.
2. As the milk cools, pour a small amount into a small non-metallic bowl, add the starter, and stir until mixed. Once the starter is dissolved, pour the mixture into the rest of the milk. Mix well.
3. Cover the bowl with plastic wrap. Then cover the plastic with a clean kitchen towel and place in a warm place for at least 6 hours and generally no longer than 8 hours. The longer you let it stand, the tarter the taste becomes.
4. Refrigerate. Use 2 tablespoons of this yogurt as starter for the next batch.

Note: Use fresh, plain, store-bought yogurt rich with active bacteria as your first starter.

Yogurt Cheese

Labni

Makes about ½ cup

Labni is yogurt drained of its water. It has the consistency of sour cream. Labni is sold in the refrigerated section of all Middle Eastern stores, or make your own.

1 cup plain yogurt

Special Equipment:
Yogurt funnel or cheesecloth

1. Spoon the yogurt into a yogurt funnel (purchased at any kitchen store), or a small-webbed strainer lined with cheesecloth, set over a deep-sided tub or bowl used to catch excess liquid.
2. Cover with plastic wrap and leave to drain for 24 hours in the refrigerator.
3. Transfer the resulting cheese to an airtight container and keep refrigerated.
4. Serve spread on bread or use as a base when preparing some of the other recipes in this collection.

Clarified Butter

Ghee

Makes 1 pound

Traditionally, Armenian cooks and bakers used clarified butter almost exclusively, particularly when frying and making pastries. It is superior to ordinary butter that contains milk solids, because it does not burn easily at high temperatures.

I've tried it both ways and found that the traditional cooks were right. Clarified butter does make a difference. Older recipes call for melting the butter, then spooning, or pouring, the clarified portion off the top of the milky bottom layer. That's okay if you possess the dexterity necessary to perform this culinary feat, but I don't, so I melt the butter then refrigerate it. As the melted butter cools, it separates.

1¼ pounds (5 sticks) butter

1. Melt the butter in a small saucepan over low heat until melted. Or melt in a microwave-safe dish in a microwave.
2. Without stirring, allow the melted butter to cool slightly before placing it in the refrigerator to harden. The clarified portion of the butter will resolidify on top and the milk solids will pool underneath.
3. When hard or almost hard, carve a hole in the top yellow layer with a knife. Drain off and discard the milky residue underneath. Continue to harvest the clarified butter by scraping off with a knife and discarding any white milky residue that remains.
4. Transfer the clarified butter into an airtight container and store in the refrigerator until needed.

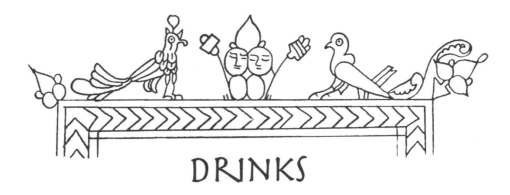

DRINKS

Chilled Yogurt Drink

Tahn

Serves 2

Tahn is especially refreshing in hot weather. It is sold, chilled in bottles like a soft drink, throughout the Middle East.

1 cup plain yogurt
1 cup ice-cold seltzer water
¼ teaspoon salt
Ice cubes

1. Place the yogurt in a deep bowl and add the seltzer water. Whisk rapidly until blended and frothy, or use a blender and whip until frothy.
2. Stir in the salt and chill with ice cubes.

Armenian Coffee

Makes 2 demitasse cups

This coffee is prepared in a small, long-handled pot tapering in and lipped at the top, called a jezvé in Turkish. Purists will grind their own coffee beans to a fine powder just before brewing. Tall, thin, brass coffee mills are sold throughout the Middle East, and in Middle Eastern stores in the United States, too.

When offering you a cup of this high-octane brew, your hostess will ask if you like it very sweet, sweet, or without sugar.

1 heaping teaspoon very finely ground Turkish or Arabic coffee
1 - 2 teaspoons sugar
½ teaspoon ground cardamom (optional)

1. Use the cup you plan on serving to measure two cups of cold water into the pot (jezvé). Add the coffee and sugar, and, if desired, cardamom.
2. Stir over medium heat. When the coffee froths up in the pot, immediately remove it from the heat until the foam subsides. Heat it again, until the coffee rises a second time.
3. Let the coffee subside again before gently pouring the top liquid off into the serving cups. There is debate about how much if any foam a good cup of coffee should have on top. I like a head of creamy foam on top. To each his own.

SWEETS

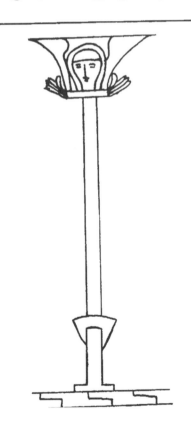

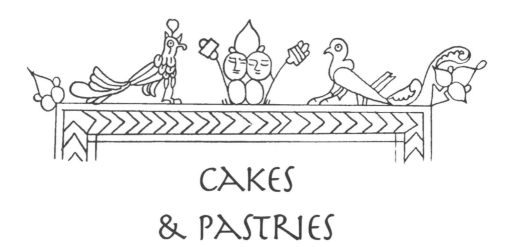

CAKES
& PASTRIES

Savory Cheese-Stuffed Kataif

Serves 12

This rich, bird's-nest-looking dessert has yummy filling options. I offer three—savory with cheese, crunchy with nuts, or totally original with chestnut and ricotta paste! Served dripping in lemony-sweet syrup, this dessert is one of the most exotic and foreign recipes in the collection.

For those unfamiliar with Middle Eastern pastries, kataif dough is simply shredded phyllo dough that looks and feels like extra thin angel hair pasta al dente. The toughest part of making this sweet may be finding the dough—an easy task if you have a Middle Eastern grocer nearby, but not so easy if you don't. Once found, this dessert assembles quickly and is fun to make and popular with everyone.

The Syrup:
1 cup sugar
¾ cup water
1 tablespoon fresh lemon juice (for a more exotic aroma and flavor, substitute 1 teaspoon rose water or orange flower water, preferably French)

The Cheese Filling: (see variations below)
2 cups part whole milk ricotta cheese
1 large egg

The Pastry:
1 pound kataif
(Apollo brand Shredded Fillo Dough [Kataif] is the easiest to find)
½ pound (2 sticks) unsalted butter, melted
¾ cup milk

The Topping:
¼ cup chopped walnuts or pistachios

Special Equipment:
1 (9-inch square) cake pan

1. Prepare the syrup first. Combine the sugar and water in a saucepan and bring to a boil. Lower the heat and simmer for 15 minutes, or until the syrup thickens. Stir in the lemon juice, and set aside to cool.
2. In a small bowl, combine the ricotta and egg. Set the filling aside.
3. Preheat the oven to 350 degrees.
4. Open the package of kataif dough and separate the strands completely in a large mixing bowl. Pour the melted butter over the dough and toss with your hands until the dough is evenly buttered. This is fun! Don't be intimidated by the dough. You can't make a mistake.
5. Arrange ½ of the dough in the pan so that it covers the bottom. Spread the filling mixture evenly over the dough. Then cover the filling with the remaining dough.
6. Cover the pan with foil and bake in the middle of the oven for 30 minutes. Remove the foil and bake an additional 30 to 40 minutes, until the top is golden.
7. Remove the pan from the oven, and while it is still hot, sprinkle the milk evenly over the entire surface, especially the edges. Cover the pastry again with foil and let sit for about 5 minutes to allow the dough to moisten.
8. Finally, remove the foil and pour the cooled syrup evenly over the top of the still-warm pastry. Garnish with the chopped nuts and serve warm.

Note: Changing the filling changes the pastry dramatically (step 2).

Variation 1: **Kataif Stuffed with Nuts**

The Filling:
2½ cups of finely chopped walnuts or pistachios
2 teaspoons ground cinnamon
Dash of ground nutmeg

Variation 2: **Kataif Stuffed with Chestnut Purée and Ricotta Cheese**

The Filling:
1 can (500 grams) sweetened chestnut purée
1 cup part whole milk ricotta cheese

Paklava

Makes 24

End any meal with a small diamond of light, not-too-sweet, layered pastry called paklava. (Baklava is the Greek name.) It is one of the simplest desserts to make—yet everyone always feels special because you did.

The Syrup:
1⅓ cups sugar
1 cup water
Juice of ½ lemon

The Pastry:
2½ cups walnuts, finely chopped
1 tablespoon sugar
¼ teaspoon ground cinnamon
½ pound (2 sticks) unsalted butter, clarified (page 230)
1 package phyllo dough (see Glossary, page 284)

1. It's important to make the syrup first, so it can cool completely before it's poured over the hot pastry. Combine the sugar and water in a small saucepan and bring to a boil. Reduce the heat and simmer until the syrup thickens, about 15 minutes. Remove from heat, stir in the lemon juice, and set aside to cool.
2. Combine the walnuts, sugar, and cinnamon in a bowl. Set aside.
3. Preheat the oven to 350 degrees.
4. Melt the clarified butter in a small bowl.
5. Remove the phyllo dough from its packaging. Cover immediately with 2 overlapping sheets of plastic wrap and a clean, slightly moistened kitchen towel to prevent the dough from drying before use.
6. Brush the bottom of the baking tray with butter. Working quickly, place 1 sheet of phyllo dough so that it fits the tray or is centered on the tray. Brush the top with butter. Repeat this process until 10 sheets of phyllo are layered in the pan.

7. Spread the nut mixture evenly over the top. Continue layering the dough as before until the remaining 10 layers are used. Brush the top with any remaining butter.

8. Carefully cut into diamond shapes with a sharp knife. Bake in the middle of the oven for 30 to 45 minutes. (Baking times will vary according to your oven and the thickness of the baking sheet you use. I recommend that the first time you make this delicate pastry, you set your timer for 30 minutes to check the pastry's progress. Continue baking until the top is crispy and an appetizing golden brown color.)

9. Remove from the oven and immediately pour the syrup evenly over the top. It's normal to hear a sizzling sound when the cool syrup hits the hot pastry and tray.

10. Cool completely before serving. Be a culinary hero—bring a tray of homemade paklava to any gathering.

✑ Tahini Paklava ✑

Makes 24

Traditionally this sweet is prepared and served during Lent. The butter-flavored cooking spray may initially not sound appetizing but the end result is absolutely mouth-watering.

The Filling:
1 cup finely chopped walnuts
⅓ cup sugar
¾ teaspoon ground cinnamon
¼ teaspoon ground cloves

The Pastry:
Butter-flavored cooking spray (see Note)
1 package phyllo dough (see Glossary, page 284)
1 cup well-stirred tahini
Powdered sugar

1. Combine the filling ingredients in a bowl and set aside.
2. Spray the bottom of the baking tray with butter-flavored cooking spray. Set aside.
3. Remove the phyllo dough from its packaging. Cover immediately with 2 overlapping sheets of plastic wrap and a clean, slightly moistened kitchen towel to prevent the dough from drying before use.
4. Working quickly, using 1 sheet at a time, place the dough in the center of your work area, the long edge nearest you. Spray with cooking spray. Repeat until 5 sheets are used. Then spoon ¼ cup of tahini about 1-inch in from the bottom edge so that it forms a ribbon approximately 1-inch wide. Then sprinkle ⅓ cup filling over the tahini strip.
5. Now fold in the left and right edges, about ½-inch. Starting from the bottom edge, fold the phyllo up and over the filling, covering it, then continue folding and rolling to the top. It will resemble a fat 12-inch ruler or jelly roll.

6. Carefully place the roll on the prepared baking tray, seam-side down. Spray the roll with cooking spray.

7. Preheat the oven to 325 degrees. Then continue filling and rolling the remaining dough until all sheets are used. You should end up with 4 (12-inch long) rolls. Cut the rolls into 2-inch lengths or 6 equal sections. Be sure to cut through to the bottom.

8. Bake in the middle of the oven for 30 to 35 minutes or until tops turn golden in color. Remove from the oven and immediately sift the tops generously with powdered sugar.

9. Transfer to a platter, and cool. Best served at room temperature.

Note: If you are not keeping to a Lenten diet, or any diet for that matter, substitute ⅜ pound (1½ sticks) unsalted clarified butter, melted. Brush butter where directed to use cooking spray.

Apricot Squares

Serves 12

In the West, the pumpkin plays a major role in holiday cuisine, but the Armenian kitchen honors the apricot. After all, the juicy, festive orange-colored apricot originated in Armenia! These squares aren't too heavy or too sweet. Served with coffee, they are just right.

The Filling:
1½ cups chopped dried apricots (about 10 ounces)
¾ cup water
⅔ cup sugar

The Cake:
¼ pound (1 stick) butter, softened
1½ cups sugar
4 large eggs
½ teaspoon vanilla extract
3 cups white all-purpose flour
1 teaspoon baking powder

Special Equipment:
1 (9-inch square) cake pan, greased

1. Preheat the oven to 350 degrees.
2. Place the chopped apricots in a medium-sized saucepan. Add the water, cover loosely, and simmer the apricots over low heat until tender, about 15 minutes.
3. Remove from heat and mash into a paste with a potato masher or fork. Add the sugar and stir until the sugar is mixed completely into the warm apricot. Set aside.
4. In a large mixing bowl, using an electric mixer, cream the butter and sugar. Adding 1 egg at a time, mix each egg into the batter for at least 1 minute at medium-high speed before adding the next egg. After the eggs have been added, the batter will be smooth and a very pale yellow color.

5. Add the vanilla and mix. Sift in the flour and baking powder. Mix until just combined.

6. Pour ¾ of the batter into the prepared pan. Spread the apricot filling evenly over the top and wave it gently into the dough beneath. Then top the apricot with the remaining batter. (I find wetting my fingers with water helps spread the dough.)

7. Bake in the middle of the oven for 45 to 50 minutes or until a toothpick inserted in the center comes out clean and the top is slightly brown.

8. Cool to room temperature before cutting into serving-sized squares.

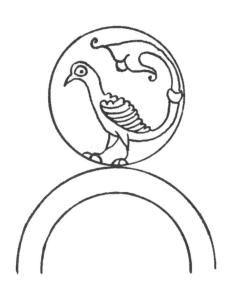

Semolina Walnut Cake

Makes 24 squares

The Cake:
½ cup semolina flour
½ cup white all-purpose flour
1 cup walnuts, finely chopped
½ teaspoon salt
¼ pound (1 stick) unsalted butter, softened
⅔ cup sugar
2 teaspoons finely grated fresh orange zest
4 large eggs

The Syrup:
⅔ cup water
½ cup sugar
2 tablespoons fresh orange juice
1 tablespoon honey
Juice of 1 lemon

Special Equipment:
1 (8-inch square) cake pan, buttered

1. Preheat the oven to 350 degrees.
2. Combine the flours, walnuts, and salt in a bowl. Set aside.
3. Beat together the butter, sugar, and orange zest with an electric mixer until pale and fluffy. Add the eggs, 1 at a time, beating well, about 1 minute, after each addition.
4. Stir in the nut mixture and spread the batter evenly in the prepared pan.
5. Bake until the top is golden and an inserted toothpick comes out clean, about 30 to 35 minutes. Transfer the pan to a wire rack.
6. While the cake is in the oven, combine all the syrup ingredients in a saucepan. Bring to a boil, stirring until the sugar is dissolved. Reduce heat and simmer until slightly thickened, about 15 minutes.

7. Pour the warm syrup over the hot cake. The syrup may initially pool on top, but the cake will absorb it as it cools. Cool the cake completely in the pan before cutting into squares or diamonds.
8. Serve topped with Wild Blueberry Compote.

Wild Blueberry Compote

Makes about 3 cups

½ cup sugar
1 tablespoon cornstarch
⅔ cup water
1 pound fresh or frozen wild blueberries
½ teaspoon rose water (preferably French)

1. Whisk together the sugar and cornstarch in a medium-sized saucepan, then add the water. Beat until smooth. Add the blueberries and bring to a boil over moderate heat, stirring. Boil, stirring, 2 minutes, then drain in a sieve set over a bowl. Set the berries aside in a different bowl.
2. Return the juices to the saucepan and simmer, stirring occasionally, until the syrup slightly thickens, about 5 minutes. Stir in the rose water, then pour the syrup over the blueberries and allow to cool.

Note: Thawed frozen pitted cherries (1 pound), including juices, may be substituted for blueberries. Sour cherries are best, if you can find them.

Glazed Walnut Cake

Serves 10

Dropping by the house for coffee and a sweet is a favorite way for friends to get together throughout the year, but especially during the holidays. Your guests will rave about this light, airy cake that, when drenched in syrup, becomes rich and nutty.

The Cake:
½ cup white all-purpose flour, plus additional for preparing the pan
1 teaspoon baking powder
¼ teaspoon salt
1½ cups finely chopped walnuts
2 teaspoons finely grated fresh orange zest
6 large eggs, separated
1 teaspoon vanilla extract
1 cup super-fine instant dissolving sugar

The Syrup:
1 cup sugar
1¼ cups water
½ teaspoon ground cinnamon
½ teaspoon orange flower water (preferably French), or
1 teaspoon Armenian cognac

Special Equipment:
1 (9-inch round) cake pan, greased and floured; shake out excess

1. Preheat the oven to 350 degrees.
2. Combine the flour, baking powder, salt, walnuts, and zest in a mixing bowl and set aside.
3. In a separate bowl, beat the egg yolks at medium speed with an electric mixer until pale, thick, and creamy. Add the walnut mixture and the vanilla. Mix well.

4. In a third bowl, beat the egg whites on high. adding the sugar, a little at a time, until the whites are firm and shiny.

5. Transfer a small amount of the egg whites to the walnut mixture and, with a wooden spoon, fold in the whites. This will loosen the pasty walnut dough. Once the dough is loosened, continue to gently fold in the remaining egg whites.

6. Pour the batter into the prepared pan. Bake in the middle of the oven for 45 minutes, or until the top of the cake is crusty. Remove the pan from the oven and cool on a wire rack.

7. Make the syrup while the cake is baking by bringing the water, sugar, and cinnamon to a boil in a saucepan. Lower heat and simmer for 15 minutes. Remove from heat, stir in the orange flower water or cognac, and let cool.

8. While the cake is still warm, turn it out from the pan to a serving plate and poke a generous number of holes in it with a toothpick. Pour the syrup along the outside perimeter of the hot cake. The cake will fall in the center and naturally pull the syrup inward.

9. Serve warm or cooled to room temperature. If serving warm, a dollop of vanilla ice cream really enhances this sweet treat. It's as good as, if not better than, an all-American apple pie.

Karakul

Serves 12

For those of us not familiar with the unique food combinations and unusual preparation techniques common outside the United States or Europe, this recipe may seem different. It is different, because I learned to make this unusual cake in Armenia. For that reason alone, it's worth a try.

7 eggs, separated
2 cups sugar, plus 2 tablespoons for topping
7 tablespoons butter
1 teaspoon baking soda
1 teaspoon white vinegar
4 cups white all-purpose flour
2 tablespoons unsweetened cocoa
1 teaspoon vanilla extract
2 cups apricot jam (use Armenian-made jam, if possible)
¼ cup sugar

Special Equipment:
1 (9 x 13-inch) cake pan, greased

1. Beat the egg yolks with 1 cup sugar in a large mixing bowl with an electric mixer. Partially melt the butter and beat it into the yolk mixture.
2. Dissolve the baking soda in the vinegar in a small bowl before stirring it into the batter. Then add the flour, 1 cup at a time, mixing well after each addition. The resulting dough will be crumbly.
3. Divide the dough into 3 equal parts. Press 1 part into the prepared pan.
4. Add the cocoa to the second part; mix well. Place the cocoa-flavored dough into a plastic bag and place it in the freezer. Place the remaining third in a different plastic bag and put it in the freezer, too.
5. Meanwhile, preheat the oven to 375 degrees.
6. With an electric mixer, beat the egg whites on high until stiff in a medium-sized mixing bowl. Then add the remaining 1 cup sugar and the vanilla. Mix well.

7. To assemble this multi-layered cake, spread the jam evenly over the top of the dough in the pan. Remove the cocoa-flavored dough from the freezer and crumble it evenly over the jam. Then spoon the stiff egg white mixture evenly on top. Remove the remaining bag of dough from the freezer and crumble it evenly over the egg white layer. Finally, sprinkle the top lightly with sugar.

8. Bake in the middle of the oven 20 minutes, or until golden on top.

9. Allow the cake to cool before cutting into individual serving squares. Serve with coffee or tea.

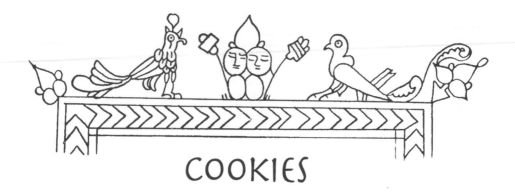

COOKIES

Almond Cookies

Makes 4 dozen

In 1915, my husband's grandmother survived the death march from her home village of Palu in central Ottoman Turkey, across the desert, to Aleppo, Syria, where she began her life again. She refused to talk about the past. Instead, she found an almond tree in the park that bloomed pink every spring like one she had been forced to leave behind. Every year after her survival until the time of her death, she broke her Lenten fast with these buttery cookies made with almonds from that tree. This recipe is her legacy of hope and redemption.

½ cup coarsely chopped almonds
2 tablespoons butter, plus ½ pound (2 sticks) butter, melted
½ cup sugar
½ cup water
½ teaspoon almond extract
1 large egg, beaten, set aside ¼ for top glaze
3 cups white all-purpose flour
2 teaspoons baking powder
½ teaspoon baking soda

1. Preheat the oven to 350 degrees.
2. In a small skillet over medium heat, sauté the almonds in the 2 tablespoons butter until golden; stir frequently to prevent burning. Drain the nuts on a paper towel and set aside to cool.
3. Pour the ½ pound melted butter in a large mixing bowl. Add the sugar, water, almond extract, and ¾ beaten egg, mixing between each addition.
4. Sift the flour, baking powder, and baking soda into the batter. Mix well, then add the toasted almonds.
5. Roll the batter into walnut-sized balls. Place the balls on an ungreased cookie sheet and press each down gently with a fork. Brush the tops with reserved egg.
6. Bake in the middle of the oven for 15 to 20 minutes, or until the cookies are golden and cracking slightly on top.
7. Remove cookies from the oven and cool on the sheet for 1 to 2 minutes before removing to a wire rack.
8. Serve anytime. These light, nutty treats store well in an airtight container.

Shortbread Cookies

Khourabia

Makes 3 dozen

A touch of blackberry brandy adds extra warmth and depth to this popular Armenian shortbread cookie.

1 cup solid shortening
¼ pound (1 stick) butter, softened
⅓ cup powdered sugar
3 cups white all-purpose flour
2 ounces blackberry brandy (see Note)
1 teaspoon vanilla extract
½ cup walnuts, finely chopped
Powdered sugar

1. Preheat the oven to 375 degrees.
2. Combine the shortening, butter, sugar, flour, brandy, vanilla, and nuts in a large bowl; mix well.
3. Roll the dough into ropes approximately ½-inch in diameter. Cut 2-inch cookies from the ropes, then gently flatten and shape each into rectangle or S-shaped cookies.
4. Arrange the cookies on an ungreased cookie sheet and bake in the middle of the oven for 10 minutes.
5. Transfer to a wire rack to cool and top with sifted powdered sugar.

Note: Substituting a strong cognac or whisky for the brandy works well, too.

Walnut Cookies

Makes about 30

Serve these original-recipe cookies as a delicious encore to any meal.

Non-stick cooking spray
1 large egg
1 cup powdered sugar, plus additional for topping
2 teaspoons baking powder
Zest of ½ lemon or more to taste
¼ teaspoon vanilla extract
2 cups ground walnuts

1. Preheat the oven to 350 degrees. Grease a few cookie sheets with cooking spray and set aside.
2. Beat the egg and 1 cup powdered sugar together with an electric mixer until combined. Add the baking powder, zest, vanilla, and ground walnuts. Mix well. The dough will form a firm but sticky paste.
3. Form small spoonfuls of dough into balls the size of small walnuts and roll in a dish of powdered sugar.
4. Arrange the powdered dough balls 1½ inches apart on the prepared sheets.
5. Bake the cookies in the middle of the oven for 15 minutes or until golden. Remove immediately to a wire rack to cool.
6. Serve with coffee or alongside a dish of vanilla ice cream topped with red maraschino cherries for a festive finish to any meal.

Tahini Cookies

Makes 4 dozen

Non-stick cooking spray
¼ pound (1 stick) butter, softened
1 cup well-stirred tahini
1 cup super-fine instant dissolving sugar
½ cup firmly packed light brown sugar
1 large egg
2½ cups white all-purpose flour
1½ teaspoons baking powder
¼ teaspoon salt
1 cup finely chopped walnuts
Red sugar sprinkles or sesame seeds (optional)

1. Preheat the oven to 350 degrees. Grease a few baking sheets with cooking spray and set aside.
2. Cream the margarine, tahini, and sugars together in a large mixing bowl with an electric mixer until light. Add the egg and beat well.
3. In a separate bowl, sift the flour, baking powder, and salt twice, then fold into the batter. Add the walnuts. The dough will not come together but will stay crumbly.
4. For best results, use an ice cream scoop to remove a scoop of dough. Roll into walnut-sized balls. Press each ball gently into a disk. Arrange the disks on the prepared baking sheets and press each disk with a fork to imprint ridges on the top of each cookie. Top with red sugar sprinkles for Valentine's Day, or sesame seeds, if desired.
5. Bake in the middle of the oven for 12 minutes or until light golden.
6. Cool the cookies on the baking sheet for 5 minutes before transferring them to a wire rack. Store in an airtight container.

Molasses-Tahini Cookies

Makes 3½ dozen

These cookies are my own invention using my husband's favorite breakfast spread as a base. They are dark in color and rich in taste.

1 cup Molasses-Tahini Spread (page 261)
¼ cup butter, softened
¼ cup solid shortening
½ cup firmly packed light brown sugar
1 large egg
2½ cups white all-purpose flour
½ teaspoon baking powder
½ teaspoon salt
½ cup chopped dates or raisins

1. Preheat the oven to 350 degrees.
2. Cream the molasses-tahini mixture, butter, shortening, and brown sugar with an electric mixer at moderate speed until light and fluffy. Add the egg and beat well.
3. In a separate bowl, sift the flour, baking powder, and salt together twice, then fold into the batter. Add the fruit.
4. Roll the dough into walnut-sized balls. Press each ball down gently with a fork on ungreased baking sheets.
5. Bake each sheet in the middle of the oven for 12 minutes. Cool the cookies on the baking sheet for a few minutes before removing them to a wire rack.
6. Store in an airtight container.

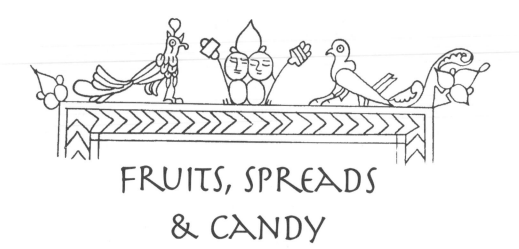

FRUITS, SPREADS & CANDY

❧ Fresh Candied-Pumpkin Slices ❧ Dipped in Chocolate

Makes 60 slices or more

Fall is pumpkin season across the United States, and this traditional Armenian recipe celebrates the fresh pumpkin in a special way. Whether picking a pumpkin to decorate with, carve into a jack-o-lantern, or cook and eat, it's best to choose one with a hard rind, a bright orange color, and a firm stem.

Starting this recipe in the afternoon of Day 1 can make the lengthy waiting times easier to live with. Pickling lime and lemon salt (citric acid) can be found at your local Middle Eastern market. You may also want to sharpen your knives; it will make the pumpkin easier to slice.

Day 1:
> ½ cup Mrs. Wage's Pickling Lime powder
> 4 quarts (1 gallon) water
> 1 medium-sized pumpkin

Day 2:

8 cups sugar
4 quarts (1 gallon) water
1 teaspoon lemon salt (citric acid)

The Dipping Chocolate:
1½ cups (12 ounce package) semisweet chocolate chips
2 teaspoons solid shortening

Day 1:
1. In a large earthen or ceramic bowl, dissolve the lime powder in the water. (Do not use a metal bowl for this recipe.)
2. Cut the pumpkin in half, downward from the stem. Clean out the seeds and stringy inner core. (Wash and set the seeds aside for toasting, page 42.) Cut the pumpkin into strips, about 2- to 2½-inches wide. Cut each strip crosswise into 2½-inch-long pieces. Peel the rind with a peeling knife. Cut each piece into ¼-inch-thick slices. This method keeps the slices crisp.
3. Put the pumpkin slices in the lime water and soak at least 12 hours (overnight).

Day 2:
4. The next morning, wash the slices well in cold running water a couple of times to make sure no lime remains. Drain and set aside.
5. In a large pot, bring the sugar and water to a boil, stirring occasionally, until the sugar dissolves. Add the pumpkin slices and cook covered for about 3 hours. The pumpkin flesh will be clear, almost translucent. Stir in the lemon salt (citric acid) at the 2½-hour mark to prevent the sugar from crystallizing later.
6. Remove the cooked slices from the sugar water and rinse under cold running water. The slices will be crisp and sweet.
7. Prepare the dipping chocolate by heating the chocolate chips and shortening in a double boiler until melted, about 5 minutes. Stir the shortening into the chocolate with a wooden spoon.
8. Dip 1 pumpkin slice at a time halfway into the melted chocolate and set the chocolate-dipped slice on waxed paper to dry.

9. Serve at room temperature alone as a fancy black and orange dessert or combine with a scoop of vanilla ice cream for a special autumn treat.

10. Stored in an airtight container in the refrigerator, the chocolate-dipped slices will keep for a few weeks.

ॐ Stewed Fruits with Walnuts ॐ

Khoshab

Serves 4

This luscious fruit compote garnished with nuts and cognac is traditionally served in celebration of the New Year or a baby's birth.

The Compote:
1 cup dried apricots, quartered
1 cup pitted prunes
1 cup raisins
½ cup powdered sugar
3 whole cloves
¼ teaspoon allspice
1 lemon, thinly sliced
1 cinnamon stick (optional)

The Topping:
Chopped walnuts
Spiced rum or cognac

1. Rinse the apricots, prunes, and raisins under cold running water and place in a large saucepan. Cover with water. Let soak, covered, about 8 hours (overnight).
2. Place the covered saucepan over high heat and bring to a boil. Lower heat and simmer for 10 minutes.
3. Add 1 cup water, powdered sugar, cloves, allspice, lemon slices, and cinnamon, if using. Continue to cook for 5 minutes or until fruit softens. Remove from heat and discard the cloves, lemon slices, and cinnamon stick. Let cool, then refrigerate.
4. Served well chilled, topped with chopped walnuts and spiced with rum or cognac. Also delicious over ice cream!

Fresh Fruit and Berries with Minted Yogurt

Serves 6

1 cup plain yogurt
1½ tablespoons honey
1 tablespoon chopped fresh mint, or 1 teaspoon dried mint
4 firm-ripe plums, pitted and chopped to bite-sized pieces
3 cups assorted berries (such as raspberries, blackberries, blueberries, and strawberries)
Fresh mint springs (optional)

1. In a small bowl, stir together the yogurt, honey, and mint. Cover and refrigerate until ready to serve.
2. Combine the fruit in a large serving bowl.
3. When ready to serve, divide the fruit into individual serving bowls and spoon minted yogurt on top. Garnish with fresh mint sprigs, if desired.

✑ Molasses-Tahini Spread ✑

Makes 1 cup

My husband grew up eating this breakfast spread as a child in Syria.

½ cup well-stirred tahini
½ cup molasses

1. Stir the tahini and molasses together until blended.
2. Serve spread on pita for breakfast.

Sesame Brittle

Makes 1 sheet

2 cups toasted sesame seeds
1½ cups dry roasted sunflower seeds
1½ cups roasted, unsalted, coarsely chopped almonds
1 teaspoon salt
1 teaspoon baking soda
2 cups sugar
⅓ cup light corn syrup
⅓ cup water
4 tablespoons (½ stick) butter

Special Equipment:
Candy thermometer (optional)
1 (10 x 13 x ½-inch) baking pan, coated well with non-stick cooking spray
Heavy rolling pin
Waxed paper

1. Combine the sesame seeds, sunflower seeds, almonds, salt, and baking soda in a bowl. Set aside.
2. In a 3-quart or larger heavy-bottomed saucepan, heat the sugar, light corn syrup, and water over medium-high heat, stirring continuously with a wooden spoon until the sugar is dissolved.
3. Bring the syrup to a boil and boil without stirring for about 10 minutes, until the hard-crack stage (300 to 310 degrees if using a candy thermometer). The hard-crack stage has been reached when a drop of syrup forms hard, brittle threads when dropped into a glass of ice-cold water.
4. Place the prepared baking pan in a warm (250 degree) oven for about 10 minutes. Warming the pan will make it easier to roll out the brittle.
5. Now stir in the butter until it dissolves, then boil without stirring for about 15 minutes until the soft-crack stage. The soft-crack stage has been reached when a drop of syrup forms hard, pliable threads when dropped into a glass of ice-cold water (270 to 290 degrees).

6. Remove the syrup from the heat and immediately stir in the nuts until all are covered.

7. Working quickly, set the heated baking pan on a flat heat-resistant work surface and spoon the brittle into the pan, cover with waxed paper, and use the heavy rolling pin to roll the candy out as evenly as possible into the pan. Work fast, but be careful not to burn yourself on the the hot pan or the hot candy!

8. Allow to cool to room temperature before breaking into serving-sized pieces. Stored in an airtight container, this brittle will stay fresh for a long time.

❧ Fig Jam ☙

Makes about 3½ cups

This jam is tasty on toast alone or with a slice of cheese.

1¼ cups sugar
¾ cup water
2 pounds firm-ripe fresh figs, peeled, trimmed, and quartered
2 strips (3 x 1-inch) fresh lemon rind
2 tablespoons fresh lemon juice
¼ cup toasted sesame seeds

1. Simmer the sugar and water in a large, heavy-bottomed saucepan, stirring, until the sugar is dissolved.
2. Gently stir in the figs, lemon strips, and lemon juice. Continue to simmer gently, uncovered, stirring occasionally, until thick and syrupy, about 1¼ to 2 hours.
3. Fold in sesame seeds.

Note: Jam keeps, covered and chilled, for about 1 month.

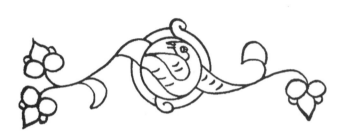

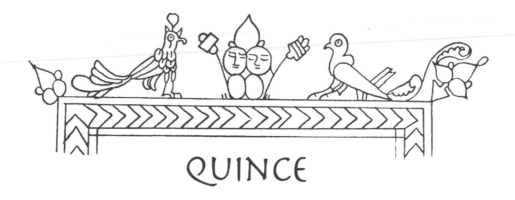

QUINCE

☞ Quince Preserves ☜

About 3 pints

Native to the Caucasus and northern Persia, the quince is a fruit with history. In Greek legend, Aphrodite successfully bribed Paris, Prince of Troy, for the quince that Eris, the Goddess of Strife, threw into a banquet crying, "The fairest shall have it!" In payment, Aphrodite arranged for the most beautiful woman in the world, Helen, Queen of Sparta, to fall in love with him—a love that sparked the Trojan War and christened the fruit the "golden apple of Discord." More recently, Biblical scholars have speculated that the Forbidden Fruit of the Garden of Eden was a quince (it's rarely eaten raw due to its rough texture and astringent flavor). The aromatic quince and epic passions have been intertwined since time immemorial.

My family's history with the fruit goes back to when my aunt and her family purchased a home with a fruit-bearing quince tree growing in the yard. Decades later, she had three trees and we nicknamed her yard "The Quince Orchard of New England." (Most of the quinces sold commercially are grown in California.)

But it was my grandmother who cared for the trees. She watched the fruit for signs of ripening during the final days of September and labored in the kitchen for days afterwards making her royal red quince preserves and jelly. After she passed away, I gladly took on the job.

6 large ripe quinces
Sugar

Special Equipment:
Self-sealing (½ pint or 1 pint) canning jars, washed and sterilized
per manufacturer's instructions
Cheesecloth

1. Wash and wipe the fuzz off the outside of the quinces, if necessary. Peel, core, and quarter the fruit. Reserve the cores and peelings in a saucepan and add cold water just to cover. Set aside.
2. Cut the fruit into thin slices and immediately put the slices in cold water to prevent discoloring.
3. Cover the saucepan containing the cores and peelings and bring to a boil. Lower heat and simmer, slowly, about 35 minutes. Then strain through cheesecloth, pressing out all the juice. Transfer the juice to a large pot.
4. Drain the quince slices before adding them to the juice. Then add just enough additional cold water to cover the fruit, if necessary, and cook over medium heat until tender, about 30 minutes.
5. Now, measure the quantity of quince juice and slices using a metal measuring cup so the hot juice will not crack it. Return the quince mixture to the original pot and add ¾ cup sugar for every 1 cup of cooked fruit and juice.
6. Over moderate-low heat, stir until the sugar is dissolved and simmer, uncovered, stirring often to keep from scorching, until the syrup reddens to a deep ruby color, about 1 hour.
7. Test the preserves for jelling by placing a small spoonful on an ice-cold plate. The liquid will thicken on contact when done. When you are certain the preserves will jell, fill small, sterilized jars (½ pint is best) and seal immediately. Properly sealed, these preserves will last indefinitely, until opened. Once opened, refrigerate.

❧ Quince Jelly ❧

Makes 24 (1 pint) jars

Clear, garnet-red quince jelly will grace your breakfast table for the coming year and make all the effort this recipe requires worthwhile.

3 grocery store bags ripe quinces
12 hard red apples (do not use McIntosh apples)
Juice of ½ lemon

Special Equipment:
Preserving kettle
2 extra-large strainers
2 jumbo-sized pots
Cheesecloth
Self-sealing (1 pint) canning jars, washed and sterilized
per manufacturer's instructions

Day 1:

1. Wash and wipe the fuzz off the outside of the quinces, if necessary. Remove the stems and any imperfect spots. Do not pare or core them. Instead, cut the fruit into small pieces and toss the pieces into a preserving kettle with enough cold water to cover.
2. Cut the apples the same way and add to the kettle. Add more cold water if necessary.
3. Cook over moderate heat, stirring from the bottom often, until the fruit becomes mushy like applesauce, about 2½ hours. Remove from heat and let cool.
4. Straining the fruit mush is most easily accomplished by lining 2 extra-large plastic strainers each with two layers of cheesecloth. Set the strainers over 2 jumbo-sized, deep pots, and pour half of the fruit mush in each strainer. Allow the fruit to drain over the container for at least 6 hours (overnight). Do not squeeze or push the liquid through the cloth. The jelly will be cloudy if you do.

Day 2:

5. In the morning, strain the collected juice again through new cheesecloth.

6. Measure (in cups) the juice as you transfer it back into the cleaned preserving kettle. Bring it to a boil and add 1 cup of sugar for every cup of juice, less 1 cup sugar (i.e., if you have 10 cups liquid, add 9 cups sugar). This will leave you with 1 cup more juice than sugar, resulting in a little less sweetness. Continue to boil; skim any scum that forms at the top and stir frequently, so the jelly will not burn. This step takes a long time—hours. The jelly will turn pink then ruby-red, then a darker almost garnet red as it cooks.

7. Once the jelly is dark red, begin dropping a small spoonful on an ice-cold plate. If it thickens up immediately, it will jell in the jars. When you think you're close, squeeze in the lemon juice and test frequently, because the color is quickly affected by too much boiling.

8. When done, remove from heat and fill the self-sealing jelly jars immediately. Properly sealed, this jelly will last indefinitely until opened. Once opened, refrigerate.

❧ Quince Paste ❧

Makes about 1 pound

Quince paste is a sweet concentration of cooked quince and sugar that is allowed to harden and then spread like a jelly or served with fresh cheese on a hearty bread as an appetizer. It is sold in gourmet shops, especially around the holidays, at top dollar, so making this delicate paste yourself is as economical as it is delicious.

Quince paste makes an excellent holiday gift for the discerning gourmands on your list.

2 pounds (about 4 medium-sized) fresh quinces
Sugar
Powdered sugar

Special Equipment:
Blender or food processor
1 (9-inch square) cake pan, sprayed thoroughly with non-stick cooking spray
Waxed paper

1. Wash and wipe the fuzz off the outside of the quinces, if necessary. Peel, core, and quarter the fruit.
2. In a heavy-bottomed pot, combine the quinces with just enough water to cover and bring to a boil over moderate heat. Stirring occasionally, cook about 30 minutes, or until the fruit is soft.
3. Pour into a blender and purée. Measure the purée with a measuring cup as you return it to the heavy-bottomed pot. At this stage the purée looks and smells like applesauce. Stir in an equal number of cups sugar as you have purée (i.e., if you have 2 cups quince purée, add 2 cups sugar).
4. Now, continue to cook, stirring, over moderate heat until the mixture turns a ruby red color and reduces to a thick, stiff consistency that pulls away from the sides and the bottom of the pan when stirred, about 30 minutes.
5. Pour into the prepared pan and let set for 8 hours (overnight).

6. In the morning, cut into squares and set the squares on a wire rack. Sift tops with powdered sugar, turn the squares over and sift again with sugar, then leave the squares to dry, about 2 hours. When dry, wrap each square in waxed paper and store in an airtight container in the refrigerator.
7. Slice and serve. This paste will keep for about a month.

Variation: ## Apricot Paste

Substitute 1 pound of dried apricots for quinces. Cook until fruit is very soft. Add 2½ cups sugar. Spread mixture in the prepared pan and sprinkle with finely chopped unsalted pistachio nuts.

Quince Coffee Cake

Makes 1 cake

Quinces are in season from late summer to early winter. They may be a tad pricey, but you only need two medium-sized fruits to make this incredible-tasting and equally eye-catching coffee cake.

This recipe is so good I recommend baking two cakes (make two single recipes); eat one and freeze the other for the holidays.

The Fruit (see Note):
2 medium-sized quinces
2 cups water
¾ cup sugar
2 teaspoons fresh lemon juice
1 stick cinnamon

The Cake:
1¾ cups cake flour
¼ teaspoon ground cinnamon
¼ teaspoon salt
¼ pound (1 stick) unsalted butter, softened
1½ cups sugar
1 large egg yolk
3 whole large eggs
½ cup heavy cream
1 teaspoon vanilla extract

Special Equipment:
1 (9-inch round) cake pan

1. Wash and wipe the fuzz off the outside of the quinces, if necessary. Peel, quarter, and core the quinces. Cut the fruit into ⅛-inch-thick slices.
2. Bring the quinces, water, sugar, lemon juice, and cinnamon stick to a boil in a saucepan. Reduce heat and simmer, stirring occasionally, until the cream-colored quince slices turn a deep ruby color. The time may range

from 1 to 2 hours. Quinces will generally darken in color the more you cook them.

3. Drain the cooked fruit in a large sieve. Cool on paper towels to room temperature. Then chill, covered, for at least 1 hour and up to 3 days before using.

4. When you are ready to make the cake, preheat the oven to 350 degrees. Butter and flour the pan, knocking the excess flour out, and set aside.

5. In a bowl, sift the flour, cinnamon, and salt together twice. Set aside.

6. In another bowl, use an electric mixer to beat together the butter and sugar until light and fluffy. Add the egg yolk and whole eggs, 1 at a time; beat for at least 1 minute after each addition. Add half of the flour mixture and all of the cream. Beat until just combined. Add the remaining flour and the vanilla. Beat again until just combined. Fold the chilled quince slices into the batter and spread the batter evenly in the prepared pan.

7. Bake the cake in the middle of the oven for 1 hour and 10 minutes, or until a toothpick inserted in the center comes out clean.

8. Cool on a wire rack for 20 minutes, then turn the cake out of the pan onto the rack to cool completely.

9. Serve with coffee, or topped with a dollop of vanilla ice cream for an extra-special treat.

Note: This cake is easiest made over a 2-day period. I usually cook the quinces a day or so before I make the cake.

Quince Linzer Cookies

Makes 2 to 2½ dozen

You cooked up a batch of quince jelly, right? Good, because now it's time to open up a jar and make some festive holiday cookies. In this recipe, I've tweaked a traditional butter cookie recipe and used my homemade quince jelly in the center. The resulting cookies taste spectacular! Plus, their bright red center will add cheer and grace to your holiday dessert table.

If you didn't make quince jelly, and can't buy it, substitute seedless raspberry or strawberry jam.

2 cups plus 2 tablespoons cake flour
½ teaspoon salt
½ pound (2 sticks) unsalted butter, softened
¾ cup sugar
2 large egg yolks
1 teaspoon vanilla extract
1½ cups Quince Jelly (page 268)
Powdered sugar

Special Equipment:
Waxed paper
Heavy rolling pin
1 (3-inch round) and 1 (1½-inch round) cookie cutters (substitute a
Linzer cookie cutter, if desired)

1. Sift together the flour and salt into a mixing bowl. Set aside.
2. Beat the butter in a large mixing bowl with an electric mixer on high speed for about 5 minutes, or until pale yellow and fluffy. The butter needs to be whipped for a long time, otherwise the batter is too stiff when chilled.
3. Add the sugar and beat at medium-high speed until very pale, about 2 to 3 minutes. Scrape down the sides of the bowl and add the egg yolks and vanilla. Beat again until blended. Add the flour mixture, slowly, until the batter collects together into a dough.

4. Shape the dough into a log. Wrap the log in plastic wrap and refrigerate for at least 2½ hours or up to 3 days.

5. When you are ready to make the cookies, preheat the oven to 350 degrees and line 2 cookie sheets with waxed paper.

6. On a lightly floured work surface, roll dough out until it is ⅛-inch to ¼-inch thick. Cut into 3-inch rounds with a circular cookie cutter.

7. Place half of the rounds on the prepared cookie sheets and spread a thin, even layer of quince jelly over each. Cut a hole in the center of the remaining 3-inch rounds with a 1½-inch circular cookie cutter so each round becomes a ring. Place a ring on top of the jelly layer to make an open sandwich cookie. (Use the scraps and the holes cut out of the rounds to make more cookies.)

8. Bake the cookies in the middle of the oven for 6 to 8 minutes depending on the thickness.

9. Cool on a wire rack. When cool, sift lightly with powdered sugar.

Quince Drop Cookies

Makes 3 dozen

Non-stick cooking spray
2 cups sifted white all-purpose flour
3 large egg yolks
10 tablespoons (1 stick plus 2 tablespoons) butter, slightly softened
1 cup sugar
¼ teaspoon salt
1 large egg white, slightly beaten
½ cup finely chopped walnuts
½ cup Quince Jelly (page 268, or apricot preserves)
Powdered sugar

1. Grease a few cookie sheets with cooking spray and set aside.
2. Beat the flour, egg yolks, butter, sugar, and salt together with an electric mixer, then knead the batter by hand until smooth. Form into a ball, wrap in plastic wrap, and chill for ½ hour in the refrigerator.
3. Remove from the refrigerator and form the chilled dough into smooth walnut-sized balls. Arrange the balls on the prepared sheets, pushing each gently onto the cookie sheet so that the bottom flattens.
4. Brush with egg white and sprinkle with walnuts. Then with the handle end of a wooden spoon, press a deep hole in the center of each cookie. Chill again in the refrigerator for 30 minutes.
5. Preheat the oven to 350 degrees.
6. Remove the cookies from the refrigerator and bake for 20 minutes, or until lightly browned.
7. Cool the cookies on a wire rack. As the cookies cool, fill the holes with jelly. Once they have completely cooled, dust with powdered sugar.

Quinces Stuffed with Walnuts in Syrup

Serves 6

The Syrup:
1 cup sugar
½ cup water
2 teaspoons fresh lemon juice

The Fruit:
6 medium-sized quinces

The Stuffing:
½ cup chopped walnuts
1 tablespoon sugar
½ teaspoon ground cinnamon
¼ teaspoon ground cloves
Juice of 1 lemon

1. Prepare the syrup first. Heat the sugar in the water over moderate heat in a saucepan until boiling. Lower heat and simmer for 15 minutes, or until it thickens. Turn the heat off. Stir in lemon juice. Set aside to cool.
2. Preheat the oven to 350 degrees. Slightly oil a roasting pan large enough to fit 12 quince halves in 1 layer.
3. If necessary, rub the fuzz off the outside of the quinces until bare. Wash and pat dry. Trim off the tops and tails of the fruit. Peel completely, then slice in half. Core each half with a sharp knife, opening up a well.
4. In a small mixing bowl, combine the walnuts, sugar, cinnamon, cloves, and lemon juice. Mix well.
5. Stuff each quince half with stuffing mixture. Arrange the stuffed quince halves, stuffing side up, in the prepared pan. Cover loosely with foil and bake for 1½ hours, or until the fruit is tender.
6. Remove from the oven. Set halves on a serving tray and immediately pour syrup over them. Best served warm, but they are tasty at room temperature also.

GLOSSARY
&
INDEX

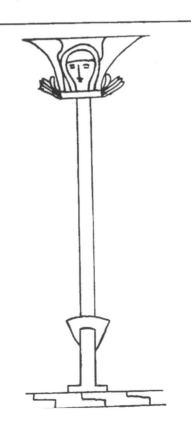

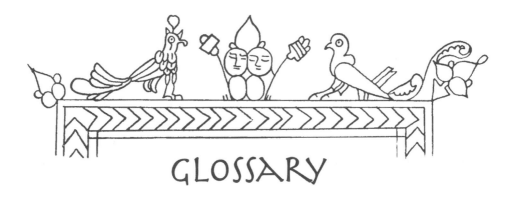

GLOSSARY

Armenian String Cheese – This cheese (tel banir) is a mild white cheese packaged in the shape of a large rope knot. It is traditionally served shredded in a serving bowl. Armenian string cheese is so popular in the United States today that it can be found in the cheese section of most supermarkets.

Arak – This is clear-colored liqueur with an ouzo-like taste. It's made in Lebanon and is readily available in liquor stores. Sometimes called "raki."

Borek – A Turkish word for pastry stuffed with a filling.

Bulgur – Cracked wheat that has been processed for Middle Eastern dishes. There are three grinds: fine (#1), medium (#2), and coarse (#3). It's sold by Middle Eastern grocers, upscale supermarkets, and gourmet stores, or can be found in your local supermarket under the Near East brand. A box of Near East Tabouli Wheat Salad contains ¾ cup fine-grain bulgur, and a box of Wheat Pilaf contains ¾ cup of coarse-grain bulgur. Discard the spice sack.

Cayenne – Ground hot red pepper. It is also known as Aleppo pepper and is sold under that name by many spice vendors.

Cumin – This spice is second in worldwide popularity to black pepper. It can be purchased at your local supermarket in powder or whole seed form. All the recipes in this collection call for ground cumin. If grinding the whole seed, adjust down the amount called for in the recipe—the ground seed gives you more flavor. The seeds grind into an olive-green-colored powder.

Dolma – Refers to a vegetable stuffed with a meat-based mixture.

Fava Beans – Native to the Mediterranean basin, these legumes resemble a large lima bean. Fava beans are popular in Mediterranean and Middle Eastern dishes and can be purchased dried, cooked in cans, and, in season, fresh.

Grape Leaves – The leaves of the grapevine. Wild grapes grow throughout the United States. Pick the young, tender lime-green leaves or buy leaves packed in brine from California in Middle Eastern stores or fine delicatessens.

Hummus Paste – The paste is composed of finely ground chickpeas and tahini. Cans of prepared hummus are sold in Middle Eastern markets.

Kasseri – This is a creamy gold-colored Greek cheese made from sheep or goat milk. Its firm texture and composition are perfect for both grating and melting. It can be bought in gourmet cheese shops and Middle Eastern stores. Substitute kashkaval cheese, also Greek, or most any sheep's-milk cheese, or try an aged provolone.

Kataif – This is shredded phyllo dough. It resembles soft, pliable shredded wheat (which can be used as a substitute). Kataif is sold in Middle Eastern stores. The most widely distributed brand is Apollo. Apollo sells a 1-pound box labeled Shredded Fillo Dough.

Kheyma – The best cut of lamb (leg or better) or beef (top round or better), trimmed of all fat (even large fat marbles within the meat), then ground three times. It's sometimes called kufteh or kibbeh meat. Any custom butcher can prepare kheyma meat, or it can be found, frozen, in most Middle Eastern groceries.

Kibbeh – An Arabic/Turkish word for a layered, one-pan dish.

Kufteh – Kuftehs are stuffed meat, either in a meatball or layered form. Ground lamb (or beef, if you prefer) is spiced, then baked, fried, or boiled in broth. Kheyma meat is always used to prepare the outer casing or crust layer of kufteh. No matter how they are prepared, kuftehs are to Armenians what hamburgers are to Americans.

Labni – Yogurt drained of its water. Also called yogurt cheese. Find in the refrigerated section of Middle Eastern stores or make your own (page 229). Yogurt funnels can be purchased at any kitchen store.

Lentils – Lentils (vosp in Armenian) are legumes and, like other legumes, are low in fat and high in protein and fiber. Lentils have a mild, often earthy flavor, and taste best when generously spiced. Adding salt slows down the cooking process, so most recipes add flavorings last. Armenian cooks use brown lentils (for which I often substitute French green lentils) and the common red lentil. Red lentils are salmon pink in dried form but turn golden and get mushy with cooking, which makes them perfect in soups and purées. The bigger the lentils, the longer they take to cook, so brown (or French green) lentils cook a bit more slowly than red lentils, but they hold their shape better. Before cooking any lentils, always rinse them in cold running water and pick out and discard stones and other foreign objects found.

Mahleb – A flavor additive derived from black cherry pits, used extensively in Middle Eastern and Greek breads. It is sold in Middle Eastern markets in small, hard chunks that look like cream-colored pebbles or already ground to a cream-colored powder. For best results, buy the chunks and grind to a powder just before use. Refrigerate to keep fresh.

Nigella Seeds – Black caraway seeds, commonly called black seeds. They have a strong flavor and are sold in Middle Eastern markets.

Olive Oil – Olive oil is a flavorful, monounsaturated oil pressed from tree-ripened olives. The flavor, color, and fragrance of olive oils can vary dramatically. Extra-virgin olive oil is cold-pressed, a chemical-free process that involves only pressure, which produces a low-acid oil. It is considered the finest of the olive oils and it's also the most expensive. I always recommend using extra-virgin olive oil for salads and cold dishes because it really enhances the flavor of the dish. After extra-virgin, olive oils are classified in order of increasing acidity. Virgin olive oil is also first-pressed but has a higher acidity. Products labeled simply "olive oil" or "pure olive oil" contain a combination of refined olive oil and virgin or extra-virgin oil. In the United States, a less colorful and flavored oil is marketed as "light." The "light" designation refers to flavor, not caloric content, as all olive oils have the same amount of beneficial fats and calories. The filtration process for this rather nondescript oil also gives it a higher smoke point than regular olive oil, so it can be used for high-heat frying whereas regular olive oil is better suited for low- to medium-heat cooking. When the type of olive oil called for in a recipe is not specified, the choice of oil is left to the cook.

Phyllo – Thin rectangular sheets of dough sold in the frozen food section of most supermarkets, approximately 20 (13 x 17-inch) sheets to a package. All the recipes in this collection are calibrated to use this size dough; however, in certain parts of the United States, the packaged phyllo dough measures 9 x 13-inches. If that's the case in your area, the recipe will make one (9 x 13 x 1-inch) pie, plus one (9 x 9 x 1-inch) pie rather than one (12 x 17 x 1-inch) pie.

Pine Nuts – These expensive little cream-colored nuts come from the large pinecones of Italy. Also called pignoli nuts. Sold in most supermarkets.

Pita – Round flat pocket loaves. Also known as Syrian bread. Find in supermarkets everywhere.

Pomegranate Molasses – A tart-tasting molasses made from the pomegranate fruit. It is sold in bottles, already prepared, in Middle Eastern and gourmet stores.

Purslane – Also spelled purslain. Called per-per in Armenian. The leaves of this low-growing ground cover or pot herb are fleshy and succulent. Find in specialty produce or farmers markets.

Quince – More yellow than green, the ripe quince resembles a large, lumpy pear. Still rock hard, its aroma is pungent and sweet, more like a pineapple and a guava than an apple or a pear. The skin is covered with downy fuzz that has to be rubbed or washed off before the fruit can be used. The flesh is a light butter-color and it's sour and astringent to eat raw, but when cooked, it softens and turns a pale pinkish-orange that deepens with additional cooking to a ruby red. High in pectin, quince is a perfect choice for jellies, butters, pastes, and preserves. Until recently, quinces were rarely found in U.S. markets, but now the season runs from August through January.

Rose Water – Rose-blossom extract. It can be found in gourmet shops or in Middle Eastern stores.

Sumac – Sumac is made from the berries of a wild bush that grows throughout the Mediterranean. It is burgundy or rust-colored and has a tangy, lemony taste. It is most often sprinkled on top of food as a condiment or garnish and is sold in all Middle Eastern markets.

Tahini – A light tan-colored paste made of ground, toasted sesame seeds and sesame oil. It has the consistency of natural peanut butter. Sold in Middle Eastern stores, health food stores, and the foreign food section of many supermarkets.

Zahtar – A thyme-like herb that is often blended with sumac bark and chickpeas or sesame seeds. Imported from Lebanon and Syria, it is sold in Middle Eastern markets.

The Traditional Healthy Mediterranean Diet Pyramid

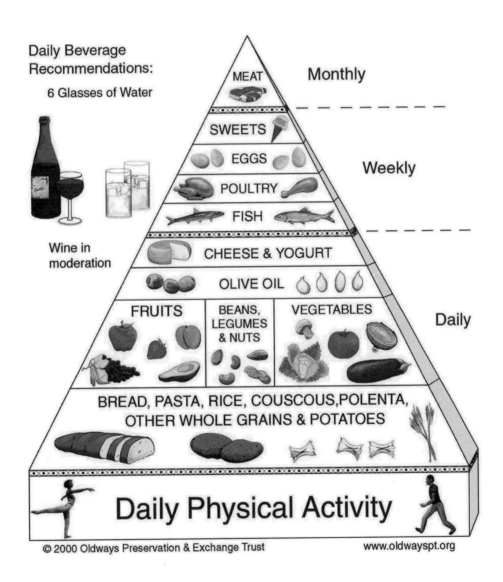

Daily Beverage Recommendations:

6 Glasses of Water

Wine in moderation

MEAT — Monthly

SWEETS

EGGS

POULTRY — Weekly

FISH

CHEESE & YOGURT

OLIVE OIL

FRUITS

BEANS, LEGUMES & NUTS

VEGETABLES — Daily

BREAD, PASTA, RICE, COUSCOUS, POLENTA, OTHER WHOLE GRAINS & POTATOES

Daily Physical Activity

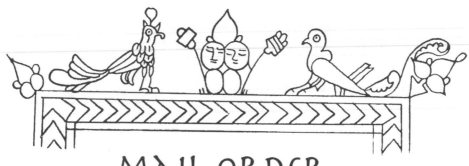

MAIL-ORDER SOURCES

Amazon.com
Gourmet Food Store
www.amazon.com

ARISA Bulgur Wheat
Sunnyland Mills
www.sunnylandmills.com

Delicacies
International Foods & Gourmet
20 Rolfe Square
Cranston, Rhode Island 02910
(401) 461-4774
Hyedeli@aol.com

Kalustyan's
123 Lexington Avenue
New York, New York 10016
(212) 685-3888
(212) 683-8458 Fax
www.kalustyans.com

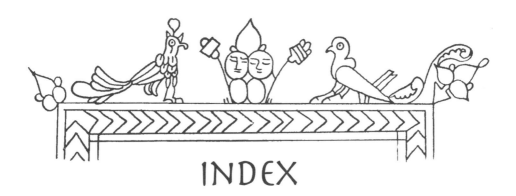

INDEX

NOTES

NOTES

NOTES